THE DOCTORS' LIVES!

THE INSIDE STORY OF THE JOURNEY AND EXPERIENCES OF DOCTORS.

ANIL CHAWLA M. D.

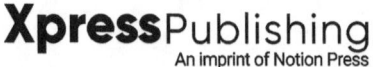

XpressPublishing
An imprint of Notion Press

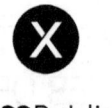

XpressPublishing
An imprint of Notion Press

No.8, 3rd Cross Street,CIT Colony,
Mylapore, Chennai, Tamil Nadu-600004

ISBN 978-1-63606-582-3

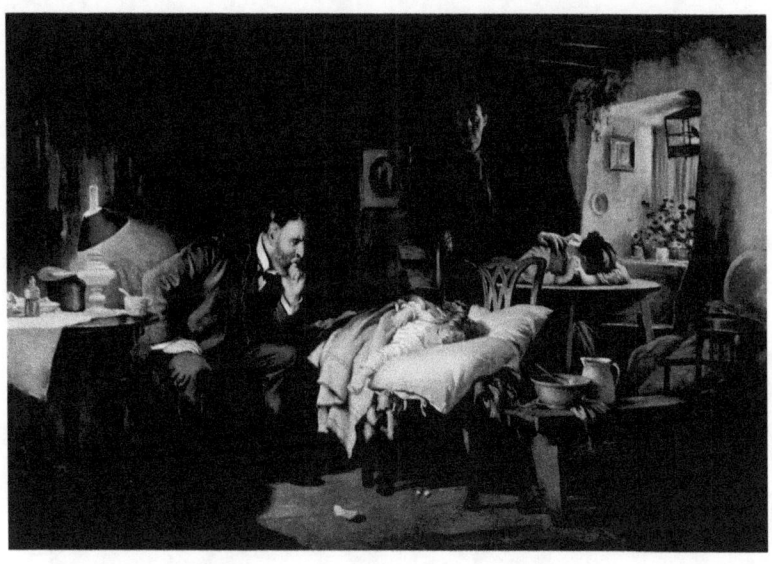

'The Doctor' - By Joseph Tomanek, reproduction of original by Luke Fildes

DEDICATION

This work is dedicated to all the Corona Warriors- the doctors and others who are fighting the war against the COVID 19 virus pandemic. Corona Virus or COVID 19 Pandemic is currently going on in the world, infecting close to twenty five million people and killing over 850,000 people. Among the killed are the doctors and nurses themselves who died while treating these patients and getting infected themselves. Doctors and nurses have been the front line warriors in this world war against the Corona Virus. Over two hundred doctors have died in India alone and in many other countries many doctors and nurses have laid down their lives serving their patients.

Beware Corona!

It is tiny, good looking one with spikes and projecting sirens,

But it is selfish to the core; it wants to proliferate its sirens!

This Corona Virus wants to live forever; others may live or die,

It may not succeed in its endeavors but it is giving its best try.

It will enter a man or woman and make them cough and sneeze,

When another one is near, they will catch the droplets in the sneeze.

The droplets are full of this tiny, good looking Corona,

It will multiply in abundance in the new host; this deadly Corona.

If you go out, be near, meet and befriend a person infected with Corona,

Corona is smiling, you are supporting Corona, saying, "Long Live Corona,"

If you thus support Corona, you are not supporting yourself or your family,

Don't support Corona, stay home support your Nation, your bigger family.

The whole world is one big family, 190 nations of the world are affected,

Corona has united the world; all regions, religions, rich or poor it has infected.

Corona is not caring; it is a monster killer, over 25 million people are infected,

Over 850,000 are dead; the planet is at grave risk: save yourself, don't get infected!

There is no treatment, no cure, no prevention, no vaccine so far,

Trials are happening to find a cure or vaccine everywhere near and far.

It is a pandemic like the 1918 Spanish Flu pandemic affecting the globe,

COVID-2019 is a similar killer, infecting and killing all over the globe.

In the absence of cure, SMS is the only rule to be followed by everyone,

Sanitizing hands, Masking and Social distancing is the SMS for everyone.

Follow Lockdown and Quarantine rules, then you are helping everyone,

Support your Government and community's efforts and be the noble one.

Doctors are the frontline warriors like soldiers on a battle field,

This battle with Corona is fought by healthcare workers in the field.

They are putting their lives on the line to save the lives of other humans,

Though not super human, they are our heroes; they are the best of humans!

-

CONSECRATION:

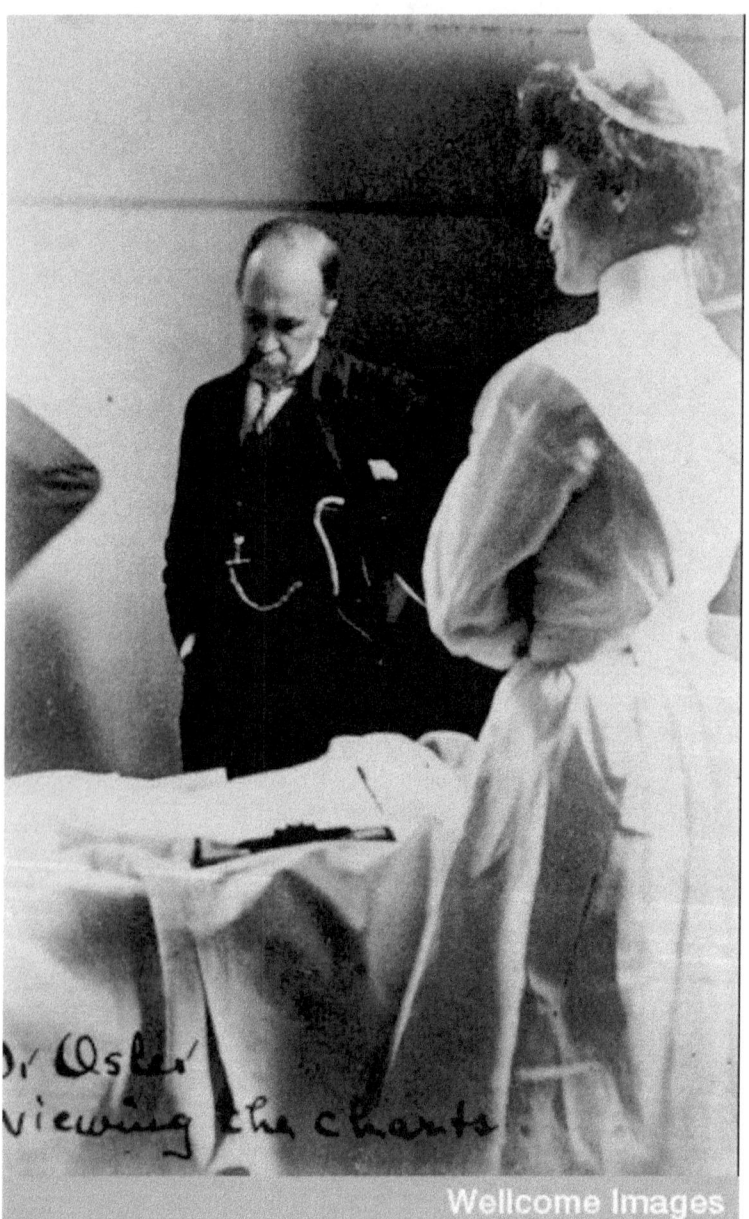

Dr Osler
viewing the charts.

Dr Sir William Osler on the ward rounds at the John Hopkins Hospital.

This work is consecrated to the memory of my ideal, Sir William Osler, the Father of Modern Medicine.

Sir William Osler, FRS FRCP was a Canadian physician and one of the four founding professors of Johns Hopkins Hospital. Osler created the first residency program for specialty training of physicians, and he was the first to bring medical students out of the lecture hall for bedside clinical training.

He was passionate about teaching and advising medical students and residents. He has written many essays/books related to this. 'A Way of Life' is one such essay which has very profound advice for medical students and young doctors in training.

His name is associated with the sign, Osler's nodes' in Infective endocarditis and also with Osler- Weber-Rendau syndrome.

His quotes are famous among medical fraternity and are often called 'Oslerisms'.

He is known as The Father of Modern Medicine. My salutations to the world teacher.!

Born: 12 July 1849, Died: 29 December 1919,

Education: McGill University- Faculty of Medicine, Trinity College School.

-

"I desire no other epitaph... than the statement that I taught medical students in the wards, as I regard this as by far the most useful and important work I have been called upon to do."

William Osler: *Aequanimitas*, "The Fixed Period" 1914:407

-

"We are here to add what we can *to*, not to get what we can *from*, Life."

William Osler

-

"One of the first essentials in securing a good-natured equanimity is not to expect too much of the people amongst whom you dwell."

William Osler

Contents

Foreword   ı   *xi*

Preface   *xv*

Acknowledgements   *xxi*

Prologue   *xxiii*

1. What It Takes To Become A Doctor   1

2. A Young Doctor In Training   41

3. Doctor: Now A Full Fledged Professional   59

4. Doctor As An Observer Of Life   93

5. Doctor Turns Philosopher   129

Author Information   157

References And Image Credits   159

Foreword

Each human being is born unique, not only in his or her unique finger prints but also in talents. Each person discovers his talent bye and bye and then needs to work on it to polish it. Then if he finds people who appreciate that talent, he finds chances to express that talent. A talent is for the whole humanity and not just for the individual to keep for himself. Some groups and organizations are talent hunters and pick up and promote individual talents. That is how society in general learns to appreciate different talents and make them live and grow.

Talents differ but that does not make anyone big or small, superior or inferior. This is expressed in the poem 'The Mountain and the Squirrel' by Ralph Waldo Emerson:

The mountain and the squirrel,
Had a quarrel,
And the former called the latter
'Little Prig'
Bun replied,
'You are doubtless very big,
But all kinds of things and weather,
Must be taken in together,
To make up an year,
And a sphere!
And I think it no disgrace,
To occupy my place,
If I am not as large as you,
You are not as small as I,
And not half so spry!
I'll not deny you make,
A very pretty squirrel track,
Talents differ; all is well and wisely put,
If I cannot carry forests on my back,
Neither can you crack a nut!"

-

Writing poetry is a talent quite different from writing prose. 'Write a Poem' published in the March 1999 issue of the Bahrain Medical Bulletin tells us how?:

'Write a Poem'

-

Writing poetry is so different from prose,
For the latter you've to think, fathom and grope,
The former just flows out, at its own will and pace,
Like from hills flows down, a river with grace.
In the twilight zone between sleep and dreams,
Or the zone between wakefulness and day-dreams,
At the drop of a hat, an idea would strike,
Then sit or lay quiet; let imagination run wild.
Words would arrange and rearrange themselves in rhyme,
A poem is taking shape; you just watch and see how it times.
Now take a pen and put it to paper,
Words will flow, you just be their jotter.
A poem would thus, come and write itself,
Once in a blue moon or daily, it will please itself,
It would create, like a brook its natural course,
A poem won't come through intention or force.
Keep your receptacle open, to get the gift of poetry,
Only you be an instrument, of this divine mystery.
A poem would then stir the heart and touch the soul,
Universal appeal is its nature, not merely a goal.
Poetry, like music is the language of the heart,
Human hearts feel and beat as one, they aren't apart.
Emotions in poetry unite mankind,
Write one such poem, feel one with your kind.
-

A poem is the creation not of the individual but of the whole universe. It is like the 'Whole in one!' May be that is true for creativity in all fields of human endeavor, talents and innovations.

The Bahrain Medical Bulletin since 1996 publishes a page which is titled, 'Talent in Medicine' and is mainly devoted to poetry by doctors. It has an initial paragraph by the Editor and it is followed by a poem or two. The Editor's paragraph, as picked up from the September 2020 issue states:

"The medical profession is not different from other workforce, sharing common interests, hobbies and talents. The majority of these activities are unrelated to medicine. Many are musicians, performers, artists, writers, critics, astronomers, photographers, etc., not to mention their excellence in the world of sports. On the other hand, there are also instances when the practice of these activities takes the form of applied interpretation of what they know in human pathobiology and the concerned function. Thus, some may be historians of clinical practice, clinical pharmacologists of locally used herbs or clinical therapists of locally practiced folk medicine. This section of the Bahrain Medical Bulletin will be devoted to "Talents in the Medical Profession" to show and exchange with others common interests and applied experience. Contributors are therefore welcomed to submit their literary works. This issue contains two poems titled "Beware Corona!" and "Even This Will Pass Away!" (The Chief Editor)

Dr Jaffar M Al Bareeq, DLO, RCP, RCS(London), Senior Consultant ENT Surgeon, who is the Chief Editor of the Bahrain Medical Bulletin, sent the following letter of appreciation when he came to know that this book was going to get published.

"Dear Dr. Anil Kumar Chawla,

We have not communicated directly through the email for awhile, but I always see you and communicate with you through your poems. Poetry has a definite role in making better and more humane physicians as it is educational to all physicians but of particular importance to our juniors and certainly to our patients. Bahrain medical Bulletin includes a page on poetry because it is not only educational but also informational that doctors have talents other than practicing medicine and that many doctors are sensitive souls and not rigid practitioners. You have been sending us your poems for over fifteen years now and I find your poetry touching and inspirational. Many of the colleagues whom I know are impressed by your poems. It is good to learn that you will be publishing your poems in a book form and you have my best wishes."

Best regards

Yours Sincerely

Dr Jaffar M Al Bareeq

Chief Editor

Bahrain Medical Bulletin - Established 1979

-

This book on the Doctors' Lives, a combination of prose, verse and art may interest doctors as well as non doctors who are interested in art and literature, in prose and poetry or verse. The author would be delighted if someone finds in it a nugget or two for use or simply a viewpoint, some information and some fun.

With grateful thanks,

Anil Chawla M.D.

Preface

PRACTICE OF Medicine is a combination of Science and Art. And there has to be a right combination of both.

If there is too much science, you may consider a patient as a machine and there is a risk of treating him inhumanely, which would defeat the very purpose of being a doctor which is to give succor and relief. And if there is only art, then any uneducated, illiterate but smart person oblivious of medical science can deal with patients like any customers and fool them for his own benefit and harm the public. That's like a quack or a charlatan.

A right mixture of science and art is essential in the making of a good and humane doctor.

Most medical schools lay emphasis solely on the teaching of the science of medicine. During their 5-6 years or longer courses there are hardly any lectures on the art and practice of medicine. Students learn a lot of scientific facts and some skills; pass their examinations and come out as doctors ready for practice.

In the field of art and practice, they are supposed to fend for themselves and basically learn by observing their seniors. The art and heart of medicine needs more attention in medical schools.

What is the art of Medicine and can it be formally taught? Teaching the art of Medicine would perhaps include bits of human psychology, sociology, morality, ethics, other humanities, language skills and a sprinkling of spirituality.

The art of medicine includes development of good inter-personal skills between human beings, one powerful through knowledge and the other sick and helpless; one provider, carer and curer and the other in need and at the mercy of his skills and benevolence. Knowledge gives power to the doctor over common human beings.

The training in art of medicine is how not to let that power go into one's head and thus not to exploit another's misery for gain and how to develop feelings of humility, kindness, devotion, readiness to help and altruism.

Doctors are respected in the community for the preponderance of such qualities and criticized for the lack of them.

With so much emphasis on Science, and grades in the science subjects as entry criteria, doctors in fact lose touch with arts and humanities even in the preparatory school before entry into medical school.

Four medical schools in the U.K. have enhanced the criteria for entry into medical school and these include not only the grades in science subjects but also assess the students' aptitude for medical practice, caring, understanding, motivation and decision making through questionnaires and semi-structured personal interviews.(1) Students good in science grades don't necessarily become better or more humane doctors.

The Medical Schools council in UK in its 2006 revised guidelines for admissions to medical schools which include besides assessing the academic record of the student several other non-academic characteristics like recognition that patient care is the primary concern of a doctor, then honesty, integrity and an ability to recognize one's own limitations and those of others, have good communication and listening skills, an ability to make decisions under pressure, to remain calm and ability to cope with stress(2).

Poetry is an art form with power to express a feeling in rhythmical form. How does it fit into the whole scheme of creating more humane doctors? Quite often a poem conveys a lot in a few words. A poem can convey human emotions and feelings in a brief span of a few lines. A poem being lyrical and musical is easier to read than a paragraph of prose on the same subject. A poem can touch the core of a being much easily and gives food for thought on human problems of existence. A poem with its use of visualization and imagination can create a spell on the reader sometimes. A poem can be meaningful and useful with guidance on practical living. For some a poem like a quote can become life changing. The brevity, rhythm, rhyme, cadence and lyrical character of a poem often make it easy to hum and sing and memorize. A poem can convey much more than an essay on the same subject which may become very verbose. Poetry is perhaps the best way of putting forth the human condition and day to day living in simple easily absorbable terms.

A doctor is the person who is in close touch with humanity and human emotions, problems, dilemmas, troubles, pains, tragedies as well as occasions of joy and happiness. People share their emotions openly with a doctor whom they often trust and consider a well wisher who will not disclose information outside nor use it for any selfish purpose. People often lay themselves bare emotionally before the doctor who has to be equally humane to empathize and help people live through their difficulties with which they came to the doctor in the first place. A doctor therefore must be good at understanding human emotions and be a good human being capable of empathy, sympathy and compassion.

In their essay, 'Healing the healer: The role of poetry in palliative care' Coulehan and Clary observe that, ' Practicing medicine with too many facts and not enough poetry leads to dissatisfaction, disappointment, and impaired healing, especially in the care of the terminally ill. Likewise, poetry deficiency cuts off an important avenue for physician self-awareness and reflectivity. Alternatively, three aspects of healing are fostered by poetry: the power of the word to heal (and also harm); the skill of "negative capability" that enhances physician effectiveness; and empathic connection, or compassionate presence, a relationship that heals without words. *Reading and writing poetry can help physicians, especially those who care for dying patients, become more reflective, creative, and compassionate practitioners.*'(3)

William Carlos Williams (4), an American Physician poet, in his poem 'Asphodel- That Greeny Flower" shows the importance of poetry in life in general by the following verse,

"It is difficult
to get the news from poems
yet men die miserably every day
for lack
of what is found there."

The teaching of humanities in medical schools in training of medical students and medical residents, to make better and more humane doctors has been the subject of a number of articles in medical literature.(5-11)

A number of medical journals include space for poetry, photography and general writings by doctors. The Annals of Internal Medicine publishes original poems under the page title "Ad Libitum" The Journal of the American Medical Association weekly presents a work of art on its cover and also publishes a poem. The New England Journal of Medicine publishes artistic photographs by doctors. The Lancet also publishes poems by physicians. Bahrain Medical Bulletin publishes poems under the page title "Talent in Medicine" in its every issue. Thus the importance of art forms and poetry in particular is being recognized worldwide as of importance for the practice of the science and art of Medicine and keeping practicing doctors in touch with the humanities.

At many medical schools such courses are already included, for example, the Stony brook University in New York runs a six week elective course for medical students called, "Becoming a better MD through Poetry" during which under an instructor poems of physician poets and general poets especially those that are medical care related, are read and recited and reflected upon. At the end of the course through which attendance is mandatory the students are assessed and may write their own poems and submit. (12)

Harold Horowitz (13) conducted an experiment to include poetry during ward rounds which included house staff as well as medical students. The considered purpose was, to see if " the process of humanizing rounds as a method to create physicians who are more caring, and perhaps alleviate the burnout that often occurs among overworked house-staff and awed medical students." Twenty of the ninety minutes of the round were kept for the purpose of reading and reciting poetry. After the end of the study period almost all participants felt they enjoyed and gained from the sessions.

Foster and Freeman (14) studied the perceptions of six General practice registrars in two poetry based sessions during the course of their vocational training. At the end of the study they concluded: "These registrars reported difficulties expressing feelings in the culture of science-based medical training. Poetry sessions may provide an environment for emotional exploration, which could broaden understanding of self and others. The participants recognized development of key skills including close reading, attentive listening and interpretation of meaning. These skills may help doctors to understand individual patient's unique experience of illness, encouraging personalized care that respects patients' perspectives."

From all of the above attempts to integrate poetry in the life of doctors at every stage of their training and careers, poetry seems to exert positive effects on their development as good and more humane doctors, developing their abilities to empathize with the patient as also to understand themselves better and perhaps in the prevention of burn-out in the middle of their careers.

Some physicians are themselves practicing the art of writing poetry while simultaneously practicing the science and art of medicine in their day to day living. Green (15) observes that, 'literature has been the favored nonmedical pursuit of physicians probably because the practice of medicine is suffused with narratives, the patient's history being one.'

Anne Hudson Jones (16) extensively investigates the number of physician poets in the history of Western Medicine and elaborates on some of the current British and American poets. She quotes an estimate by Daniel Bryant about the percentage of American physician poets to be 0.0019 since 1930 (17) thus showing the rarity of this combination of the two arts of healing in one person, one for the body and the other for the mind and spirit. As mentioned earlier the trend of physician- poets is increasing as some Medical journals are regularly publishing poetry of the current physicians.

Poetry and Medicine may seem related in only an indirect way to us but the Greeks kept both arts under the same god Apollo, their god of the sun (16). The data on other countries having such physician poets is lacking but sure the art that touches humanity and human spirit must be alive and well elsewhere too.

This work by a doctor, on doctors contains a mixture of expressions in both prose and verse.

References quoted are detailed in the end of the book.

-

Anil Kumar Chawla
MD (Internal Medicine), MRCP (UK), FRCP (Glasgow)
Global Hospital and Research Center,
Mount Abu, Rajasthan, India. 307501.

-

-

Sir William Osler on significance of arts and poetry for doctors:

-

"While medicine is to be your vocation, or calling, see to it that you have also an avocation – some intellectual pastime which may serve to keep you in touch with the world of art, of science, or of letters."
William Osler, _Aequanimitas._ 'After 25 years' 1904:213.

-

-

"Nothing will sustain you more potently than the power to recognize in your humdrum routine, as perhaps it may be thought, the true poetry of life – the poetry of the commonplace, of the plain, toil-worn woman, with their loves and their joys, their sorrows and their griefs."
William Osler: _Aequanimitas_ 'The Student Life' 1914:413.

Acknowledgements

I am grateful to all my teachers who inspired me to speak, to write, to excel.

I am thankful to all my friends who always bucked me up along the journey.

I am thankful to all my patients who gave me an opportunity to listen to them, observe and serve them.

This work would not have taken shape but for the great co-operation and persuation from my family of three doctors- wife Shashi, a medical doctor and daughter Aditi and son Aman, both Doctors of Philosophy or PhDs.

I also thankfully acknowledge the creators and distributors of the images used in this book. The individual image credits are duly given in the chapter in the end.

I am thankful to Notion Press, the publishers of this book, without whose help at every stage, this daunting task could not have been completed.

I am indebted to all.

Prologue

The book is divided into five sections:

Chapter I: What it takes to become a doctor?
PART A: Preparing to enter medical school.
PART B: Enters medical school.
Chapter II: A Young Doctor in training.
Chapter III: Doctor, a full Professional now!
Chapter IV: The Doctor as an observer of life.
Chapter V: The Doctor turns Philosopher!
INDEX

CHAPTER I: WHAT IT TAKES TO BECOME A DOCTOR
PART A: PREPARING TO ENTER MEDICAL SCHOOL
FIRST STEP: ONE DREAMS TO BE A DOCTOR
Dream, dream, dream!
DREAM MUST BE FULFILLED NOW
Come On, Do It!
PREPARE WELL: STUDY EFFICIENTLY
SQ3R
HARD WORK OUT OF LOVE
Love will do!
NO FEAR. FOCUS: PERFORMANCE
Focus: Performance!
MEDICINE IS A SCIENCE: YOU ARE A SCIENCE STUDENT
Lessons in Science
INSPIRATION AND MOTIVATION IS NEEDED
Fly High!
TRY, TRY AGAIN
The threshold!
JOINING GROUPS PREPARING FOR ENTRANCE TESTS
Tools!
CHAPTER I
PART B: YOU ENTER MEDICAL SCHOOL
The Mantra!

THE FIRST YEAR: THE ANATOMY HALL
Where has gone life?
LEARNING, LEARNING AND MORE LEARNING:
LEARNING ABOUT THE MACHINE CALLED MAN
Man; The Machine!
WHAT IS LEARNING IF NOT FUN
Laughter, the best medicine!
LAUGHTER IS THE BEST MEDICINE, BUT SMILE WILL DO
Smile-just do it!
LIVING IN THE HERE AND NOW
This day, this moment, That's all!
HAVING A HOBBY HELPS
Music, O Music!
THE ART OF COMMUNICATION
Speak up!
PASSING THE FINAL MBBS/MD EXAMINATION
Win the MBBS/MD Game!
NOW HAPPY TO BE A DOCTOR
The Doctors Club!
CHAPTER II
A YOUNG DOCTOR IN TRAINING
Close encounters of Clinical kind!
TAKING RESPONSIBILITY
Responsibility!
THE GROWING PAINS OF TRAINING
Post Call Zombies!
RESEARCH- THE BEGINNINGS
Curiosity!
Creativity!
MAKING A DISCOVERY IS POSSIBLE
Discover, O man!
RESEARCH WRITING
On writing a scientific paper!
GAINING WISDOM
Quotations on the wall!

CHAPTER III:
DOCTOR: A FULL FLEDGED PROFESSIONAL NOW
A Professional's job!
LEARNING IS A CONTINUOUS PROCESS
Learning all the time!
WHAT ARE THE EXPECTATIONS FROM THE DOCTORS
Great expectations, great demands!
HOW DOCTORS FEEL PRACTICING THEIR PROFESSION
Our (Doctors') Lives!
DOCTOR PATIENT RELATIONSHIP
The doctor-patient relationship!
PATIENT FIRST
Doctor: An advocate too!
ABERRATION OF THE SACRED RULE
Betrayal of trust!
DOCTOR: PRACTICE WHAT YOU PREACH
The Puffing Docs!
WHEN A PATIENT VISITS A DOCTOR IN THE HOSPITAL
A patient's patience!
PATIENT NEEDS ADMISSION
The Hospital Bed!
LISTEN TO ME DOCTOR
Can't feel my pain? Please listen to me doctor!
FAITH: FAITH IN THE DOCTOR
Faith first; life next!
WHAT IS A DOCTORS FAITH? BE GOOD; DO GOOD
My goodness!
CHAPTER IV:
DOCTOR AS AN OBSERVER OF LIFE
POVERTY AND HEALTH
Poor man's health: Who cares?
OLD AGE AND CARE ISSUES
Our elderly: Who cares?
THE CHALLENGE OF CARING FOR ELDERLY WITH
ALZHEIMER'S DISEASE

Watch your elderly!
CHILDREN ARE PRECIOUS
The Children's rights!
OBESITY AND HEALTH
Folds of Fat: Adiposa Excessiva!
Fuel watch!
Lose! Lose!
O Waist!
HAIR, BEAUTY AND HEALTH
Mysterious hair!
DOCTOR, THERE IS TOO MUCH GAS IN ME
The gas factory!
HEART HEALTH: ANGINA PECTORIS
Angina: Stable to Unstable!
ALCOHOL AND MAN'S HEALTH
O Ethanol!
DRUG ADDICTION IS KILLING: STAY AWAY
No, No, No; say No to drugs!
ROAD TRAFFIC ACCIDENTS AND THE DOCTOR
Dangerous Moves!
MAN AGAINST MAN
Road Rage!
CHAPTER V:
DOCTOR TURNS PHILOSOPHER
THE SAD STORY OF MAN
Vulnerable man!
God's Favorite
Gone in a moment-The Japanese Tsunami
WITNESSING DEATH
Till death do us apart!
THE BEGINNINGS OF NEW LIFE
Our common origins!
BREATH IS LIFE
The other umbilicus!
THE CYCLE OF LIFE

From one cavity to another!
WHAT IS MAN?
Intel inside!
THE INVULNERABLE SPIRIT OF MAN
That's the Spirit!
A DOCTOR IS FOR THE WHOLE WORLD
Beyond this and that....
UNITY OF MANKIND
A&E
Diversity is from Unity!
UNITY IS PRIMARY; DIFFERENCES SECONDARY
Innocence lost!
Wish to be a child again!
LAST WORD

WHAT IT TAKES TO BECOME A DOCTOR

All over the world, of all the professions the longest that takes to churn out a doctor is the medical profession. Perhaps rightly so, because this is the only profession that makes you capable of dealing with the health and lives of human beings!

-

To gain entry in to a medical school is the first struggle and pain that a young aspiring student has to go through. There is so much national competition to gain a spot. Students have to cram a lot of stuff to win those competitions or to get into the list of selectees. They have to study day and night in a much focused manner to ensure success in this endeavor. They have to perfect their methods and techniques of study.

-

FIRST STEP: ONE DREAMS TO BE A DOCTOR!

-

You dream of becoming a doctor day in and day out for years together and also work for fulfilling this dream. For years on end you don't forget your dream. You keep reminding yourself of your dream lest it may be lost sight of. Consistency and perseverance, focus and performance are then added to the dream so that in a given time it gets fulfilled.

-

-

Dream, dream, dream!
Dreams of a bright future, some young dreamers dream;
They dream with open eyes, use all senses to dream.
A distant goal they visualize, becomes their lasting dream,
It goads them through life, until they've realized their dream.
'Dream,' they say, 'we must', for our prosperity and progress,
Imagine where would we be, with no dreamers amongst us?
Day dreaming is not enough; we must be steadfast and tough,
Work hard and persevere to make our dreams of real stuff.
"If we can dream it, we really can do it."
Such an exciting motto, some brilliant people keep.
No wonder then, we have been to the moon and back,
What ages ago we dreamt we have it now for fact.
"Dream, O dreamer dream", this is the age of dreams,
Let Science and Technology be your dream-team.
The impossible dreams of yesterday,
Within easy reach shall seem!
"I have a dream", be courageous; say it boldly,
Being a doctor is for mankind, feel it very soundly.
Team up with other dreamers for mankind's future,
Together we can make our dreams come true and prosper!

-

-

P.S. Post Script or Personal script:

The author was in class IX in high school when he first wrote on the door of his room, 'I want to be a doctor'. So the dreaming starts early. In the many years long journey to the fulfilment of the dream, one often forgets or loses sight of the goal, it is then that the family, particularly parents remind you and buck you up. Not only that, they arrange for you a corner in the house for your deep study, tell your siblings not to disturb you, arrange special group classes for you and often transport you too. So one remains indebted to one's parents. Thank you family!

-

-

DREAM MUST BE FULFILLED NOW!

-

It is never enough just to dream. A dream must be fulfilled and it requires constant flow of inspiration and hard work over a long period of time to see the dream take shape into reality. On the way lot of attractions and temptations come but one foregoes all of them and single mindedly works towards the fulfillment of the chosen dream. It requires a lot of character to remain consistent without getting bored or fed up.

-

<u>Come on, do it!</u>
There is something you wish you could do?
You see yourself in the doctor's shoes, don't you?
Day and night you wish you could do it too?
Dreams are now taking your daytime too?
Then what is it that's keeping you back?
Some fear you may not be up to it lad?
Hesitation, reluctance, doubts; the whole lot?
These are the enemies you must first kick out.
Think of just the thing you want to go for,
With full faith then you go for it; you've to go far!
Come on and start, take the plunge, dear,
Take to the field, don't watch from afar.
Once you get in the ring, you will often fall,
Take falls easy; falls are the way to get tall.
Start doing things seeming tough and intricate,
Doing alone shall reveal the secrets of the trade.
Sitting at the edge who-ever could cross a river?
Get ready and jump in, you will swim to the shore.
Do things step by step but do them you must,
Not doing, only talking won't gain you stature or trust.
Doing is the way you learn things that must be done,
Once you've done it a few times it can't be undone.
Practice with perseverance will take you a long way,
It may take you beyond your dreams in the Milky Way!

-

-

P.S. The author read a book, The law of Success by Napoleon Hill. On top of every page of that book, one line written is: 'You can do it if you think you can' and there is a poem that is inspiring. It is called, 'Thinking' by Walter D Wintle. This poem had been verbatim remembered by the author and on an occasion recited among colleagues and seniors.

-

THINKING!
If you think you are beaten, you are;
If you think you dare not, you don't.
If you'd like to win, but you think you can't,
It is almost certain you won't.

If you think you'll lose, you've lost;
For out in this world we find
Success begins with a fellow's will
It's all in the state of mind.

If you think you're outclassed, you are;
You've got to think high to rise.
You've got to be sure of yourself before
You can ever win the prize.

Life's battles don't always go
To the stronger or faster man;
But soon or late the man who wins,
Is the man who thinks he can!
https://www.goodreads.com/quotes/1033193-if-you-think-you-are-beaten-you-are-if-you

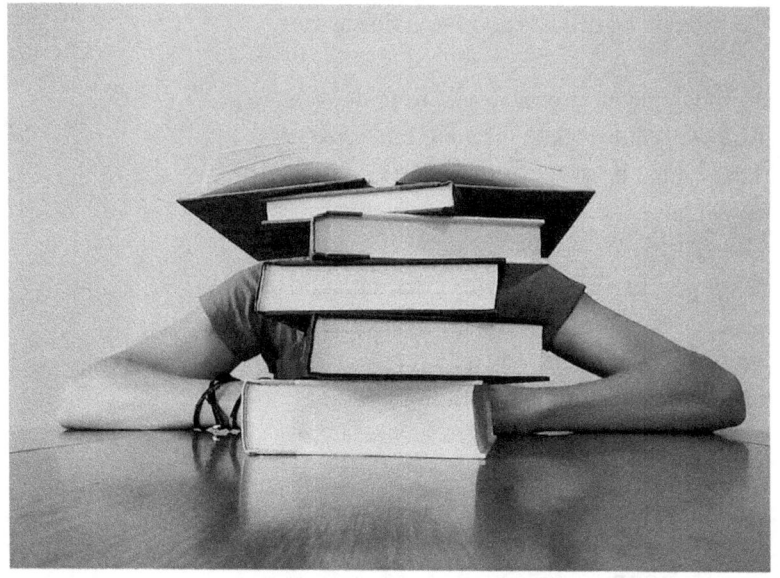

A student in the Library!

PREPARE WELL: STUDY EFICIENTLY

To pass the tough competitions, study methods have to be learnt and re-learnt and fine tuned and revised to gain a high level of efficiency. One has to solve problems a thousand times. One has to examine previous years question papers and study accordingly and widen the net of knowledge. And one of the quite useful methods of effective study propounded by many is the SQ3R.

SQ3R

So much to learn so many facts to store,
Every day brings in new facts and some more.
Small little brain, knowledge is vast and galore,
Squeezing all of it in is no small chore.
Faced with a patient a doc has no books, no notes,
So the doc must have learnt every fact by rote.

Mere rote in this matter doesn't take one afar,
Systematic learning is good practice by far.

Memorizing facts is always hard to do,
Especially for docs as facts are endless too!
There must be a way to efficiently do it by heart,
If you have the will there is a way don't lose heart.

S: survey quickly the chapter that must be learnt,
Q: then ask relevant questions, enhance involvement.
R: now read with rapt attention and an open mind,
R: recite what you read with lips open or entwined.
    Revise is the last R of this magic SQ3R,
First revision should be at the earliest hour.
Second revision can follow a week or more apart,
Things learnt this way, Sir don't easily depart.
    This SQ3R formula has helped students over the years,
Hard task becomes easy, learning becomes a pleasure.
If there is one best way of doing everything,
Try SQ3R, for knowledge is a powerful thing!
-
-

P.S. The author when he was preparing for the entrance examinations, came across a book called, 'How to Study' by fry, Ronald W. The formula SQ3R was learnt from there and applied.
-

HARD WORK OUT OF LOVE!
-

Needless to say it is years of hard labor of love which the student engages in to get into his dream profession. Hard labor should not appear or become a burden. Hard labor follows naturally if one starts to be in love with one's subjects. You can't be detesting studying something and become proficient in that. So love of your subjects is a primary input also.
-

<u>Love will do!</u>
Someone asked me once the secret of success,
"I just love my subject, that's what I guess."
"Love conquers all', you've heard I suppose,
It's true, it's true; just try and you'll know.
Love works wonders, it engulfs your brain and heart,
The subject you love permeates your every thought.
Day in and day out you think and dream of your love,
Your mind is saturated with the subject that you love.
You don't then need to force yourself to work hard,
Labor of love flows naturally you don't need a rod.
Love emanates fragrance, you can't hide or buy or sell,
Your love of the subject Sir, your enthusiasm will tell!
Your love becomes a force that pulls to it success,
Success comes to stay with you, you don't need a harness.
Just love is enough, dear come on and just love,
All else follows; you just fill yourself with love.
For once try love!

-

NO FEAR. FOCUS: PERFORMANCE

-

Fear spoils everything. Once you love your subjects, let not fear of any kind enetr your mind. Let your focus be your performance. Bring the focus back to perforrmance. No fear. 'Fear is the only foc to fear', hear O dear!

-

<u>Focus: Performance!</u>
"There aren't any spectators, no judges, just you and your bar,
Be focused on perfection; let your performance be the star."
So said *Nadia's coach to the Olympics' tiny gymnastic star,
She got bags full of gold and became a Universal Star!

"Your best work is done, when 'I am doing,' that feeling is lost;
So said a sage and how right had he taught.
We spoil everything by bringing in fear of bad results,

That fear spoils performance and leads inevitably to bad result.

We seek quick credit, immediate boost and enhancement,
We are afraid of failure, people's criticisms and disenchantments!
Fear of saving face, detracts from focus on performance,
Caught in the web of fear, who can give a sound performance?

Let's get rid of our fears, shift focus from result to performance,
To act well is our right; result is in the realms of His Benevolence!
The results are multi factorial; one known input is our performance,
Can't look after the unknowns, can take good care of our performance!

That way, we'll save ourselves from anxiety and apprehension;
Freed from fear of failure, our performance may touch perfection.
Let's begin to enjoy our performance, let other gains be a bonus,
We'll be happy in the present; leaving tomorrow to its onus!

- Nadia Comaneci, Romanian gymnast, Olympic multi gold medalist with perfect 10 scores in 1976 Olympics when she was only 14 years of age. On her a movie was made in 1984.

  -

  -

P.S. The author made a Christian Cross in front of his study table while preparing for the entrance exams. This meant that you have to work hard to the extent of crucifixion. And some couplets that pushed him to work hard were:
MITA DE APNI HASTI KO AGAR TU MARTABA CHAHE,
KI DANA KHAK MEIN MIL KAR GHUL-E-GHULZAR HOTA HAI.
Meaning : Let your individual entity be destroyed if you want perfection in anything, because the seed gets destroyed in the earth before it becomes the flower of a garden. Thus, don't try to save yourself from intense hard work.

SURKHURU HOTA HAI INSAN THOKREN KHANE KE BAAD,
RANG LAATI HAI HINA PATHAR PE PIS JANE KE BAAD.

Meaning: A man shines after stumbling and falling many times; just like hina or mehndi or henna gives its true color only after it has been crushed and rubbed on the stone.

MEDICINE IS A SCIENCE! YOU ARE A SCIENCE STUDENT.

You have to love science, to be a doctor. You have to love biology- the science of living beings and have deep desire to know the science of human body. A doctor has to have a very scientific outlook. Science is asking questions and finding answers as opposed to simply believing what is told. Science is exploring and finding out for oneself and then directly knowing. Science is fascinating and scientific outlook is a prized possession for anyone, especially a doctor.

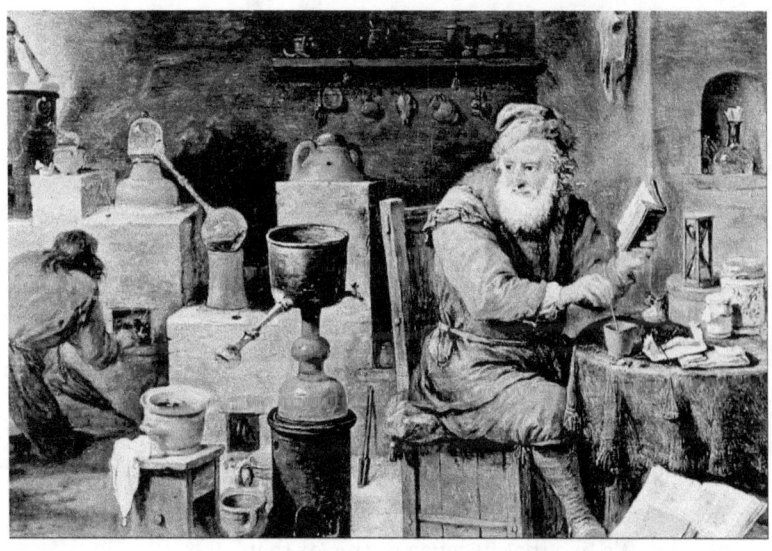

The Alchemist. Painting by David Teniers the younger, between 1640 and 1650Observation, experimentation, measurement, inference-that is Science!

-

<u>Lessons in Science!</u>
"Twinkle, twinkle little star,
How I wonder what you are?
Up above the sky so high,
Like a diamond in the sky."
This cute little nursery rhyme Sir,
Was the first lesson in science for the toddler!
The child shall now look up and around,
In wonderment make an observation sound.
'Observation' dear is the first step of science,
On this edifice is laid the structure of science.
Remember Newton? He observed an apple's fall!
From this he discovered gravity and its laws for us all.
But most of us are not like Isaac Newton,
We too observe and wonder but stop there often.
Or we accept weird explanations of the phenomena,
And carry on with our busy, hectic, mundane drama.
An observation must lead to a further step,
Why and how must stir our thought process.
Bringing up a 'Hypothesis' is Science's second step.
To prove or disprove this will be the step ahead.
For this purpose an 'Experiment' must be set up,
A well-set experiment then is Science's third step.
In an experiment measurements are made,
And these are recorded in a meticulous way.
It's these measurements then that will decide,
Whether the hypothesis was wrong or right!
The experiment can be repeated by anyone anywhere,
Measurements can be double checked by native or foreigner.
"I think it's like that because of this or that,"
That is one's subjective feeling, not a fact.
The aim of science is to remove subjectivity,
Experiment brings in objectivity and certainty.

Once in an experiment measurements are made,
From the measurements the 'results' are laid.
And its time now to draw an 'Inference'
Inference happens to be science's fourth step.
Through the inference the results of the experiment speak,
This is then knit up with the available fact sheet.
'Conclusions' are drawn; facts and myths are set apart,
This is an experiment's final but not science's final stop.
One experiment leads to another hypothesis and experiment,
The march of science this way goes on and on without deterrence.
We do end up having more and more of little, little facts,
The knowledge thus keeps piling up in books on library stacks.
No experiment? No measurement? No, that's not science!
What can't be measured is philosophy not science.
What revolves around measurements that is Science,
What changes hypothesis to fact or else, that is Science!
What's closer to Truth, open book for all - that is Science!
-

INSPIRATION AND MOTIVATION

In the difficult periods of preparation for entrance in to a medical school, the pressure is too much; the work load is even more. One needs to keep oneself motivated and inspired to keep on working towards the higher goal. No lagging behind the targets and goals. Then one seeks sources of inspiration and motivation to buck oneself up and pull oneself up from a sagging morale and tell oneself, 'Buck up'

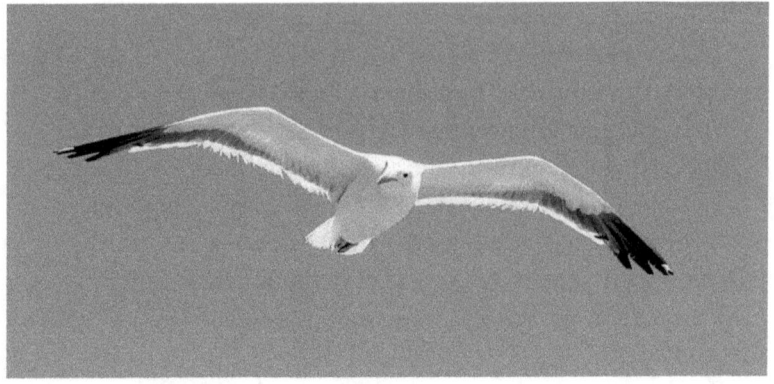

Fly High!

Fly High!
You see birds flying high in the sky,
Eagles and Seagulls fly high then dive.
Food on the ground is in their eyes,
For food it is they dive from the highs.
Some among them are of different make,
They fly high for fun and for flying's sake.
Food is not the mere goal they keep,
Flying to perfection is what they seek.
Jonathan*, a Seagull, was one such bird,
Of a tender age and a short wing-spread!
Flying was his soul and that he loved,
Small of frame, Goliath in spirits instead!
Morn or Eve when friends went hunting,
For hours and hours he kept on practicing.
Higher and higher everyday he was flying,
Heavenly bliss he found as new skills he was trying.
Some among us are just like Jonathan,
They love their jobs and work to perfection!
Hard work for them is fun, labour of love and satisfaction,
It's they who find happiness here and now in action!

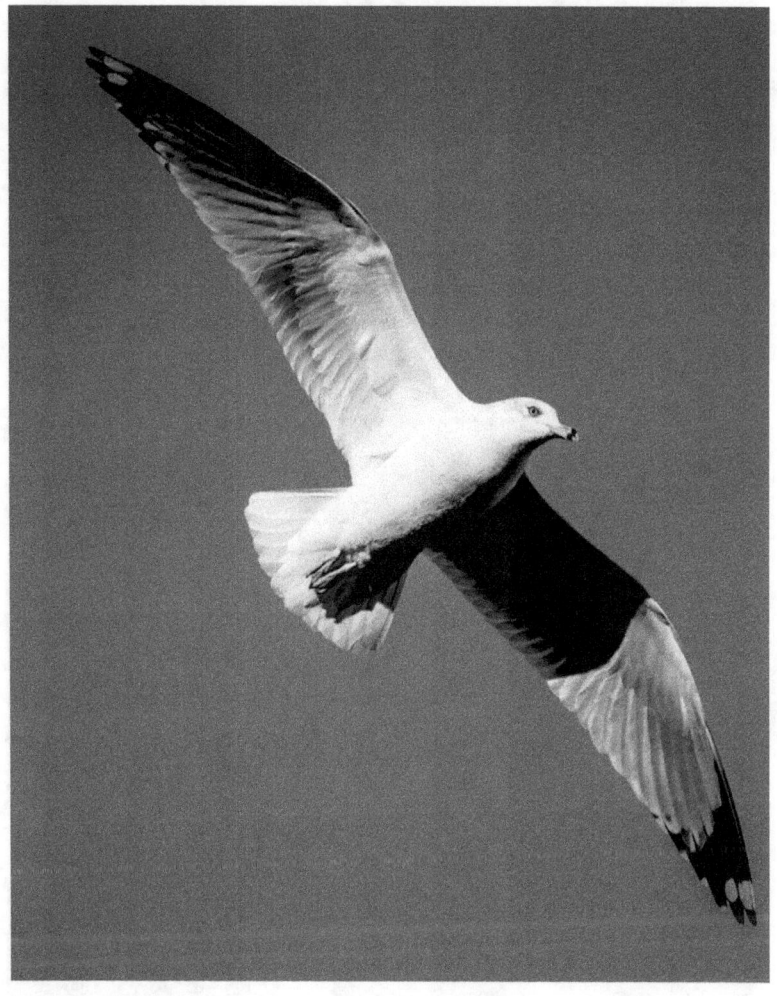

Let sky be not your limit!

*Jonathan Livingstone Seagull – a book by Richard Bach-Macmillan Publishers, USA

-

-

P.S. The author found the above very small book very inspiring.

TRY, TRY, TRY AGAIN

Another principle which motivates students is the principle of trying again and again and not give in easily to failure. The story of King Bruce and the spider is very inspiring, wherein after many failures when King Bruce was disappointed he sees a spider falling 7-8 times and each time rising and trying again till he makes it. The principle behind trying again and again is that there is a threshold or an entrance gate for success in each field and until you reach that threshold you should not quit.

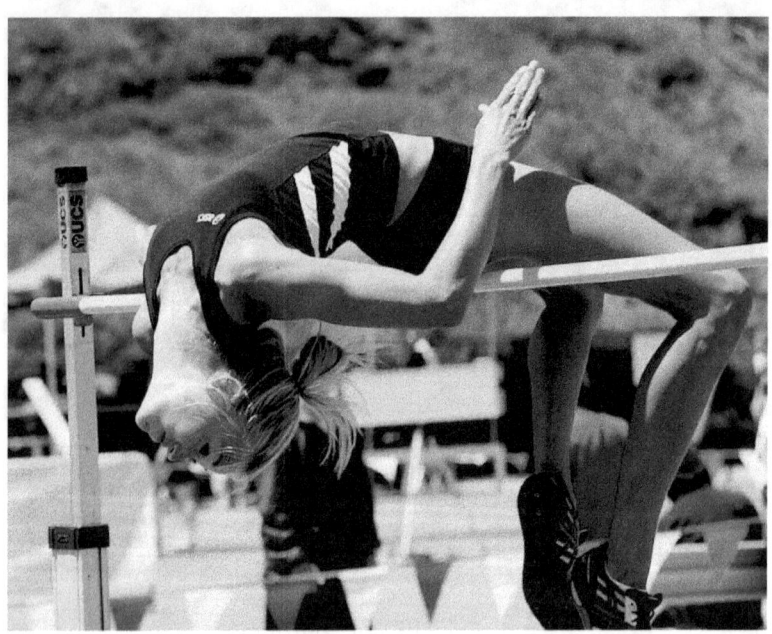

You can do it if you think you can!

The Threshold!

You want to learn something but you fail,
You tried so many times but to no avail.
You try and fail and fail until you reach a 'threshold',
Once you cross that threshold, perfection will hold.
Take swimming; you try on the shallow pool without gain,
To pick up a stroke, but flounder again and yet again.
Until one day, the trick simply, quietly dawns upon you,
Breathing easy with moving legs and arms now exhilarates you.
Take cycling; to hold the handle straight itself was a task,
For days on end you tried, the handle turned despite your grasp.
Until one day it dawns to hold the handle lose and not tight,
And then just a finger keeps it straight without a fight.
Take a mathematical problem you've been trying so hard to solve,
From daylight until it is dark; till you are about to lose your resolve.
And then suddenly there is a 'give way',
The threshold is crossed and Lo! Eureka! the problem is solved.
Take anything, you wish that badly to learn, master or do,
You practice and fail, you practice and fail and fall you do.
If you get disheartened and abandon before the threshold is reached,
You'll end up a failure dear; perseverance is what you need to succeed.
Just push a little, persist a little; press a little and a little more,
You never know when you may reach the threshold's door.
And then a light knock will let you through that esteemed door,
You'll reach success you hankered for; for days or months or more.
It's that easy, that simple; and its true for any chore,
You keep trying, keep trying and then try a little more.
The knack will dawn on you; the trick will soon be yours,
So until you reach the threshold; try that little more!

P.S. The author reminded himself to try a little more and a little more till the target was achieved by reciting the following couplet:

SAMUNDAR USEEKA TARAFDAR HAI, KAVI HAATH MEIN JIS KE PATWAR HAI,

WO KIS KAAM KA JO ADHURA HO KAAM, NA SUSTAO JAB TAK NA POORA HO KAAM.

Meaning: The ocean helps those brave boatmen who have rowing pedals in hands; what is the use of a job half done; don't rest till the job is complete and done.

JOINING GROUPS PREPARING FOR ENTRANCE TESTS

Entrance to medical school is not easy anywhere in the world. There is a huge competition for limited seats. Knowing this, preparation starts years in advance and joining group training is the norm. It is important to have a dream and be motivated and to work hard for its fulfillment. But one must use appropriate other inputs for success in this venture. So most students join group training programs for preparations for the entrance test and they start doing it a year or two or more in advance. That is called using the appropriate tools for success in any venture. With the right tools, succeed of course you will.

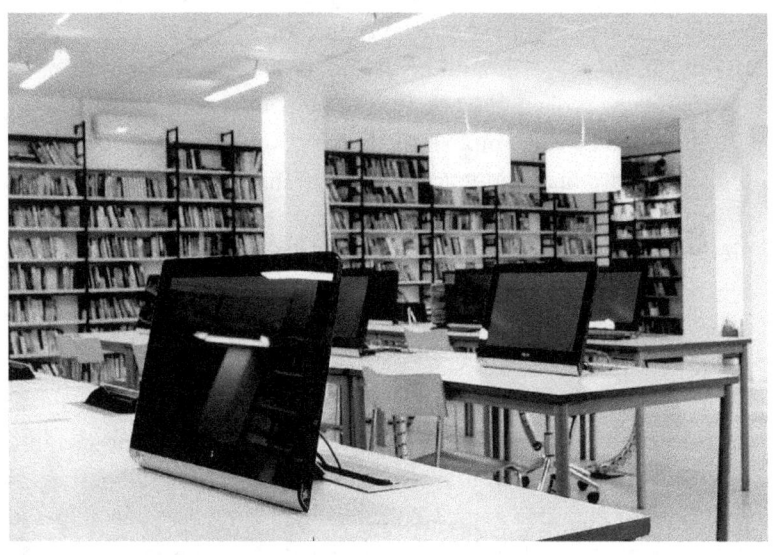

Go for right tools for success!

-

<u>Tools!</u>
"Nothing is impossible", did you hear that?
You didn't believe it, but it's a fact!
Man is endowed with so much power,
He can materialize things which were there never.
"If we can dream it, we can do it", ever heard of that?
Yes, members of GE Company, take it for a fact.
Our creativity is limited only by our imagination,
If only we can dream, we can then create and fashion.
Once you have the right desire and a fervent dream,
You are stuck on it, come rain, storm or stream.
All you then need is to lay hands on right tools,
Look for right instruments, hunt for right tools.
It's only with right tools that you can give your dreams a shape,
It's with right tools you can change the future as well as fate.
With full faith and proper training you apply these tools,

Your dream will start to turn real, you won't be fooled!
Tools, tools, tools, dear get the right tools,
You can move the mountains if you have the right tools.
Create new tools if need be for the new job,
Right tools can accomplish the hardest, toughest job.
So if you are mad about achieving anything, yes anything,
You have within the power; don't doubt about this one thing.
All you need then is to lay your hands on right tools,
You can achieve anything, dear if you have the right tools!

-

CHAPTER I: PART B : YOU ENTER MEDICAL SCHOOL

Oh My God! I have done it. We got in. There is quite a lot of natural excitement when your dream comes true. So you got into a medical college and you are so happy. But the real game begins now. How to play this game? Your teachers come to your help and guide you from Day 1. There is of course going to be a continuation of the formula of hard work and love of subjects, but then there is another feature which enters and that is of active participation at every stage of learning and training and this was told by *our teacher* in the beginning itself.

-

"No bubble is so iridescent or floats longer than that blown by the successful teacher."
William Osler. The Pathological Institute of a General Hospital. Glasgow Med J. 1911 Nov; 76(5): 321–333.

-

The Mantra
"What's the secret of your success?" someone asked,
"Interest in my subjects", I replied in quick breath.
Thinking it was a great answer better than hard work,
For hard work follows naturally, if interest is robust!
But there was "the mantra", another important reason,
Which everyone in the class should have very well known!
This "Mantra" a teacher gave the first day to the whole class,
Some of us grasped it solidly and maybe some let it pass.

This anatomy teacher, we called him Dr. C,
Dr. C told us in his very introductory speech,
To actively participate in all activities of the class!
And then he left, God bless him and his Class!
There were two or three of us who sat in the front,
Always, without fail, we got our seats without argument.
Whenever a teacher asked a question, our hands went up,
We'll rattle out the answer with energy and aplomb.
Within a few months most teachers knew us,
We were the good students among a hundred in the class.
Now we'll raise our hands but the teacher won't ask,
He wanted to give a chance to those at the back of the class.
But to keep raising our hands we had to go prepared,
Sitting in front also helped us concentrate and absorb.
Thus we participated actively whenever in class,
Our results and teachers encouraged us to stay on the top.
Friends now you know the "Mantra" Dr. C gave the class,
It's called "Active Participation", so simple, yet marvelous!
It changed our lives and brought out our best,
We gained a lot and our friends gained no less.
-

THE FIRST YEAR- THE ANATOMY HALL
-

In the medical school, besides Physiology and Biochemistry we have anatomy as a subject in the first year. In the first year in the very first class you encounter the anatomy hall where dead bodies are laid on the tables for us to dissect and learn. We take weeks and months to go over each part of the body, part by part, with the help of teachers and dissectors- the guide books for dissection.. Sometime some thoughts cross the mind- this body is there, looks intact, athletic and well built too, but there is no life in it. Where is life? What is life?

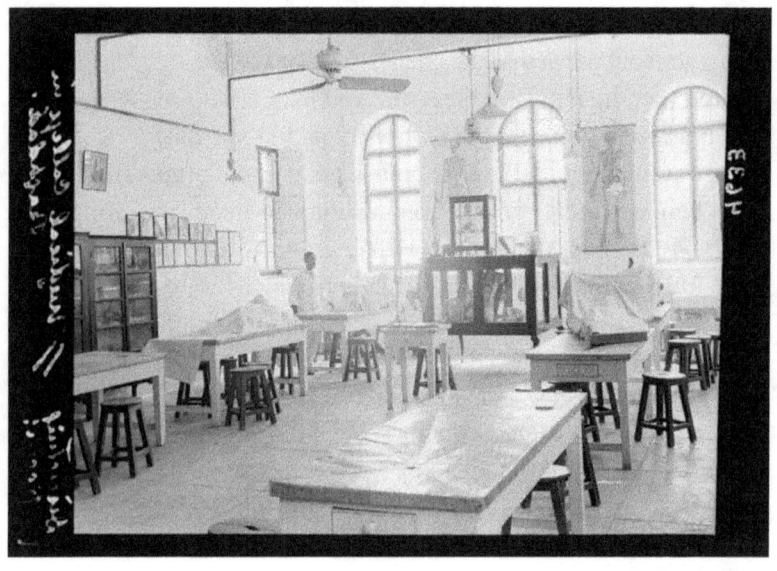

The Anatomy Hall

-

"I am firmly convinced that the best book in medicine is the book of Nature, as writ large in the bodies of men. You remember the answer of the immortal Hunter, when asked what books the student should read in anatomy – he opened the door of the dissecting-room and pointed to the tables."

William Osler: The natural method of teaching the subject of medicine. *JAMA* 1901;XXXVI (24): 1673–9.

-

<u>Where has gone life?</u>
It was a dead body that lay on our table in the hall,
Six of us* stood around it to fathom the mystery of us all.
We dissected it meticulously, step by step, part by part,
By the end of one and half year we knew it by heart.
The body is now dead, as there is now no life,
The brain and the heart are intact but dead without life.

In the cells the cytoplasm is there but where is life?
This body like another couldn't survive without life.
No-body can survive, be alive without life,
All our bodies are alive only because of life.
When life goes away, the body can be disposed away,
When life is in place; the body jumps and sways!
What moves you is life, what moves me is also life,
Life is here, life is there; what moves, well that's life!
In all of us alive, born and dying alike, is it many or one life?
Life, O Life! Tell me; are you so many or one life?
"Like one electricity lighting millions of bulbs,
Like one Sun that reflects the same in a million water pots,
Like the so many waves that arise from one sea,
Like the air that pervades inside and out, are you just one life?"
The body, made of earth (food), water, heat, air and space,
This body made of matter decays and dies after its course.
The course is set by Life as it enters the body or as it leaves,
The dead body doesn't say 'I' for 'I' is now the missing Life.
*Us: first year medical students in the Anatomy hall.
-

-

LEARNING, LEARNING AND MORE LEARNING
-

There is so much new to learn, so much information to absorb, it is simply mind blowing. Which muscle is attached where on a particular bone, how does the heart function, what kind of pathology happens to the lungs, what drugs work where and on which system, what are the diseases of various systems of the body and how to treat and manage conditions etc etc, the list is almost endless. Five plus years of learning and training makes you a bare minimum basic doctor and there is a lot further to go in specialization.
-

-

-

LEARNING ABOUT THE MACHINE CALLED MAN

As the doctor is increasing his knowledge of man's body through systematic study of subjects like anatomy, physiology, biochemistry, pathology, pharmacology, systemic medicine and surgery etc, he finds the human body to be more like a machine, a modern day computer or a robot. The science of robotics is copying the humans in every way. Man is indeed a wonderful machine. On a lighter vein, one doctor asked his car mechanic how come your fee is more than my fee! The car mechanic promptly replied, "Sir, here we have a new car model every year and we have to be up to it. For you, it is the same model since centuries!" The doctor kept mum listening to his profound eye opener reasoning.

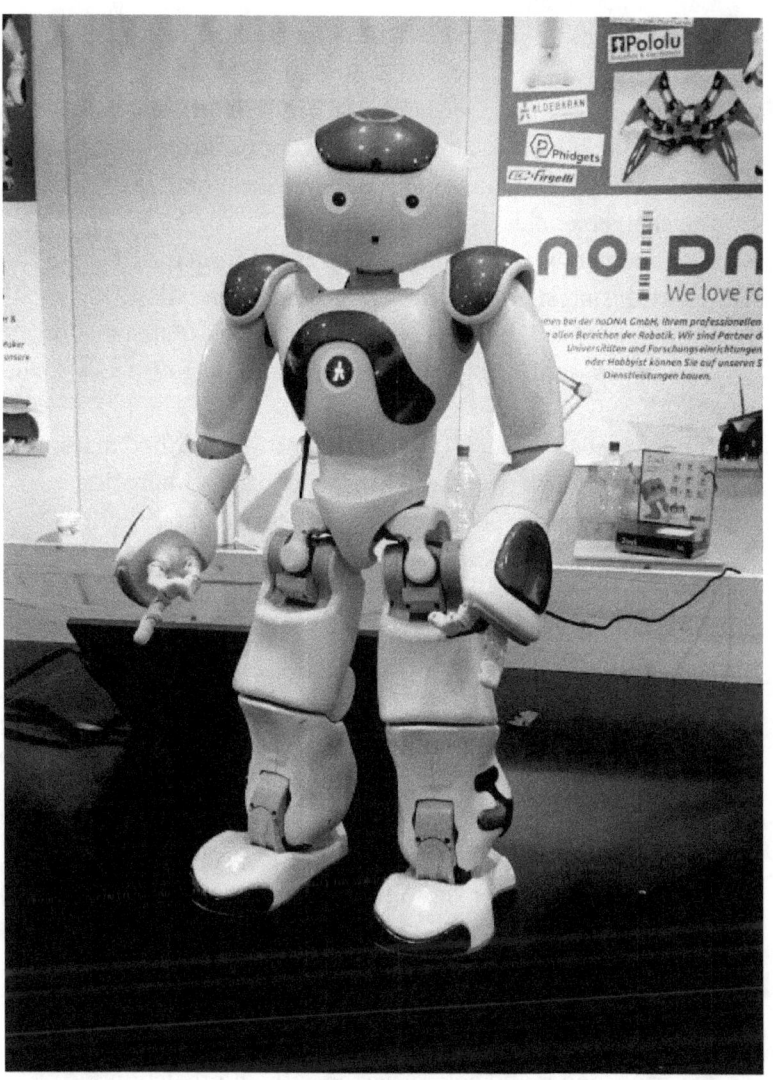

Nao_Robot_ Robocup 2016

Man: The Machine

A machine like our home PC, this one is called Man,
It has hardware, software, CPU, ROM and RAM.
There are data input, output, a VDU and a scan,
So also durables, consumables and energy demands!
The hardware is made of exo and endo-skeleton,
The skull box holds the microchip, the CPU in the Brain.
The innumerable nerves are the wires out from the CPU,
They transmit signals to the remotest parts and the VDU.
The software is of muscles, vessels and nerves of automation,
Data input occurs through vision, audition, touch, taste and olfaction.
Energy needs are met by Oxygen inhalation and food ingestion,
Output is through speech, writing, action and elimination.
Besides the Auto-mode, there is scope for voluntary action,
CPU generated will, can initiate motion and contraction.
Its VDU, the face, depicts data with varied emotions,
Its unlimited RAM and ROM create infinite combinations.
This machine can do not just calculations or locomotion,
It can also infer, guess, plan, conclude and create reaction.
Nerves with transmitter chemicals and hormones cause connections,
For such a sophisticated machine we have complex actions.
This machine, this Robot responds in ways you can't guess,
It may kick and box or show great affection and give a caress.
It may tap the feet to music, sing, and sway the head or dance,
It may jump and jog or give a joyous, naughty glance.
This machine is well stocked with inbuilt emotions,
Of happiness, sadness, anger, fear, jealousy or dejection!
Its varied moods and colors change without prediction,
To handle it is an art that few have mastered to perfection.
You can't deal with it the very way you please,
Introduce yourself with Hi, Sir, Ma'am, Smile and Please!
Wait a second for its reaction, if you want some peace,
Once the greeting is reciprocated, you may then proceed.

The only machine that man didn't make, that is Man himself,
So intricate, complex and stupendous, yet perfect in itself!
It works and works, day in and out, for years on end,
For this wonder of wonders, the credit is to its Maker, my friend.
This bipedal, mobile, functional piece of architecture, this Man,
This thinking, feeling, planning, inferring robot Homo sapiens!
This marvel of a machine only a Divine Creator could make,
Sun, Moon, Stars, Seas, Rivers and weathers who made!
Abbreviations used: PC= Personal computer, CPU- Central Processing Unit,
ROM= Read only memory, RAM= Random Access Memory,
VDU= Visual Display Unit

-

WHAT IS LEARNING, IF NOT FUN

-

You learn best when you are not under any kind of stress. You learn best when you make learning fun and add fun to learning. In the medical school, there are enough structured fun activities with student participation. There are Annual sports day competitions, annual or more frequent cultural events, student body elections, membership of committees etc. Then there are fun activities among friends which are often unstoppable except close to the exam when everybody gets in to their den. Some professors also have a jovial attitude. Once our professor of psychiatry was taking ward rounds. One patient told him he can't swallow; the professor replied, 'OK, we will get you a new head.' To this the patient laughed. The problem was anyways psychological. In every issue of the famous magazine, 'The Reader's Digest' there is one page for jokes and its title is, 'Laughter, the best medicine' Humor certainly has a great part in the art of medicine and helps in healing the mind at least.

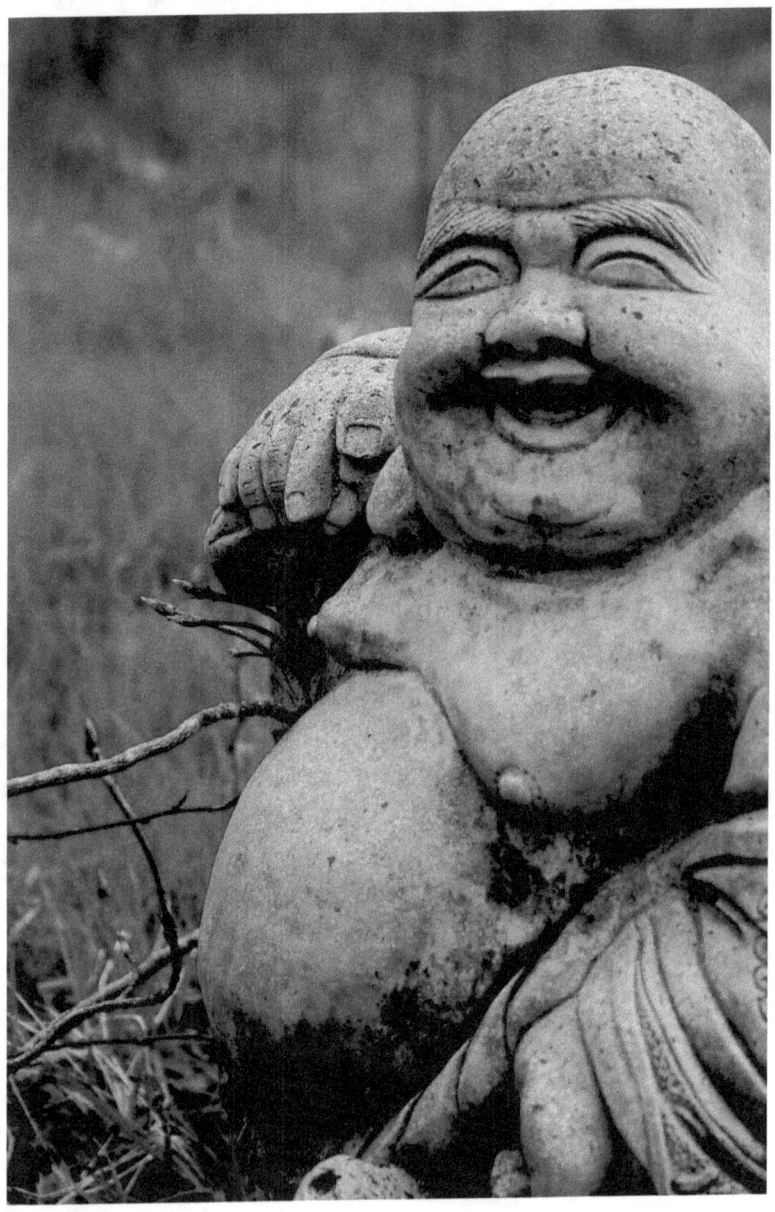

The Laughing Buddha is a great inspiration to have fun.

-

"Like song that sweetens toil, laughter brightens the road of life, and to be born with the sense of comic is a precious heritage."

William Osler: 'Two Frenchman on Laughter', CMAJ 1912(II):152

-

Laughter, the best medicine

When you're sad and depressed you need giggling therapy,

When you feel down and out you need hearty laughter therapy.

When lectures of wisdom fail you need action comedy therapy,

When you take life too seriously you need musical comedy therapy.

Life is a comedy if you looked at it properly,

There's a comedy at every corner if you looked queerly.

Here everyone looks and behaves so jeeringly,

Fire of comedy is in every heart but sparks sparingly.

Never look at life straight, you'll find a poker face,

Always look at it from an angle you'll see its bubbly face.

Never talk straight if you must elicit a smile,

Always talk upside down to bring laughter for miles.

One Mr. Q while talking kept a serious face,

His words were loaded we couldn't help but guffaw in grace.

His take on daily observations was so funny and sharp,

They were designed and meant to make you smile and laugh!

He always respected his wife for he didn't want to die too soon,

If she didn't win the argument, she'll always bring the broom,

He always said yes to her to keep trouble at bay,

He made her believe he only loved her, no one else in his way.

She wanted and he obliged; always danced to her tunes,

For she kept all the keys to his happiness and his dreams!

Their life was so happy, full of compromises and adjustments,

Mr. Q always compromised while she stuck to her embankments!

There's a funny angle to every relationship on earth,

But husband-wife is the funniest relation on planet earth.
Comedy lies hidden in human interactions of every sort,
Why men and women take life seriously, not a clue I've got!
-

-

P.S. The author came across and learnt by heart a nice poem on the value of laughter in life. The poem is called:
'Solitude' by Ella Wheeler Wilcox.
-

Laugh, and the world laughs with you;
Weep, and you weep alone;
For the brave old earth must borrow its mirth,
It has sorrow enough of its own.
Sing, and the hills will answer;
Sigh, it is lost on the air;
The echoes do rebound a joyful sound,
But shrink from voicing care.
Rejoice, and men will seek you;
Grieve, and they turn and go;
They want full measure of all your pleasure,
But they do not need your woe.
Be glad, and your friends are many;
Be sad, and you lose them all,—
There are none to decline your nectared wine,
But alone you must drink life's gall.
Feast, and your halls are crowded;
Fast, and the world goes by.
Succeed and give, and it helps you live,
But no man can help you die.
There is room in the halls of pleasure
For a large and lordly train,
But one by one we must all file on
Through the narrow aisles of pain.
-

-

LAUGHTER IS THE BEST MEDICINE, BUT SMILE WILL DO!

-

You are becoming a doctor and your job will be to cheer people up and take them across difficult times, allay their apprehensions and sometime make them smile, so they can forget their troubles. For this you yourself have to be easy on smile and smile often. As the saying goes: 'Frequently laugh and often smile; when you laugh, your troubles are half, and when you smile, your troubles reconcile' and another one says,' Laugh and the world laughs with you; weep and you weep alone. For this brave old earth must borrow its mirth, it has sorrow enough of its own.' So, smile:just do it!

-

"But whatever you do, take neither yourselves nor your fellow-creatures too seriously. There is tragedy enough in our daily routine, but there is room too for a keen sense of the absurdities and incongruities of life, and in the shifting panorama no one sees better than the doctor the perennial sameness of men's ways."

William Osler: *The Reserves of Life*. St. Mary's Hospital gazette 1907;13:95-8

-

<u>Smile, just do it!</u>
If you can't with great ease laugh or smile,
If it takes a great effort for you to smile,
If you feel it is useless to giggle or smile,
Get checked up, for you can't go far without a smile.
You may be good in your work, sincere and all,
You may get good results and laurels befall,
But nothing shall avail and nothing will prevail,
If the smile goes missing, nothing prevails!
You can't smile because you're absorbed with self,
You can't smile for you take life as serious stuff.
You can't smile for brooding it is you can't give up,
You can't smile as you think you're some alien 'pin-up'.
If you can't smile, dear you can't kick away stress,
If you can't smile, see how disappointments will press.

If you can't smile, worries may take home and rest,
If you can't smile what's the use of so-called success?
If you can smile, you needn't know any other language,
If you can smile, you needn't be rich, smart or great.
You may enter anyone's heart direct and straight,
With your smile you create human unity that's no 'fake'.
Smile to 'you' is a gift from heavens-
Did you see a donkey smiling at someone?
You better use your smile or else you'll lose it,
As over the years you see the donkeys have lost it!
Smile is a cool breeze from your heart,
Come on share it with all, you're Nature's part.
Smile: don't be a miser; it won't cost you a lot,
Smile, smile, smile, it'll lift your very own heart!

-

'Don't worry, be happy', a song beautifully rendered by Bobby McFerrin can be heard at

https://www.youtube.com/watch?v=d-diB65scQU

-

LIVING IN THE HERE AND NOW

-

A doctor must learn early not to take disappointments to heart, not to brood over mishaps of life for there will be many. If he keeps guilt in his heart about the past, he cannot move further freely and at good speed. He must keep freeing himself of the events good or bad quickly and must acquire the knack and art to do that. Then only he can keep himself stress free. Life has to be lived day to day, hour to hour, minute by minute. And the doctor must keep his mind always fresh and make it a habit to live in the present moment.

-

"The future is today, there is no to-morrow! The day of a man's salvation is now – the life of the present, of today, lived earnestly, intently, without a forward-looking thought, is the only insurance for the future. Let the limit of your horizon be a twenty-four hour circle."
William Osler. 'A Way of Life'. 1913:19

-

"No dreams, no visions, no delicious fantasies, no castles in the air, with which, as the old song so truly says, "hearts are broken, heads are turned."

William Osler. 'A Way of Life'. 1913:19

-

"Now the way of life that I preach is a habit to be acquired gradually by long and steady repetition. It is the practice of living for the day only, and for the day's work."

William Osler. 'A Way of Life' 1913:23

-

"Shut off the past! Let the dead past bury its dead. So easy to say, so hard to realize! The truth is, the past haunts us like a shadow."

William Osler.'A Way of Life'. 1913:29

-

"Many a man is handicapped in his course by a cursed combination of retro- and introspection, the mistakes of yesterday paralyzing the efforts of to-day, the worries of the past hugged to his destruction, and the worm Regret allowed to canker the very heart of his life. To die daily, after the manner of St. Paul, ensures the resurrection of a new man, who makes each day the epitome of a life."

William Osler. 'A Way of Life'. 1913:32

-

"Live neither in the past nor in the future, but let each day's work absorb your entire energies, and satisfy your widest ambition."

William Osler. Aequanimitas 'After 25 years'. 1914:213

-

"Shut out all of your past except that which will help you weather your tomorrows"

William Osler

-

<u>This day, this moment, that's all!</u>
Each day I get up and out of my bed,
I'm born again, I am new and fresh.
There's new awareness, mind is free of encumbrances,

I'm ready to face the world, let it throw challenges.
I make it a point to enjoy what I do,
Be it tough tasks or simply going to the Loo!
I love smiling and I love every moment,
I love what life is giving me moment by moment.
Why should I complain and spoil my mood?
I don't accumulate grievances to cause a bad mood.
I let go of the last moment as the past moment,
So I can stay fresh in this one, the only real moment.
When the past impinges on my consciousness-
I don't get lost in its thoughts; don't let them make a mess.
If it arises again, I don't get tired of burying it again,
It doesn't attract or trap me; I keep awake in the now again.
When the day dreaming about the future starts,
I am aware of it and don't in imagination get lost.
I bring my attention back every time into the present moment,
I don't want to lose it, I love this very moment.
A visual cue sometimes draws me away from this moment,
An auditory stimulus may get me on a ride away from the
moment.
A cloud from the memory arises, on it I fly away from this
moment,
If I am unaware I stay away, else I bring myself back to this
moment.
In this moment I'm breathing and I love it,
In this moment I'm alive and I love it.
I'm thankful and grateful for the gift of every moment,
This gratitude makes me smile; I love just this very moment.
-

P.S. The author learnt by heart in his college days, the following
couplet:
"Happy the man and happy he alone,
He who can, call today his own.
He, who secure within can say,
Tomorrow do thy worst, for I have lived today."

--

-

P.S. The one short story that bowled me over............" Tanzan and Ekido, two Zen monks were walking along a country road that had become extremely muddy after heavy rains. Near a village they came upon a young woman who was trying to cross the road, but the mud was so deep it would have ruined the silk kimono she was wearing. Tanzan at once picked her up and carried her to the other side.

The monks walked on in silence. Five hours later, as they were approaching the lodging temple, Ekido couldn't restrain himself any longer. "Why did you carry the girl across the road?" he asked. " We monks are not supposed to do things like that."

"I put the girl down hours ago," said Tanzan. " You are still carrying her?"................

Source: Page 139, " A New Earth" by Eckhart Tolle, the author of "Power of Now"

-

HAVING A HOBBY HELPS

-

A doctor has to develop in to a balanced person in whom head and heart work synchronously. That will make him a better and more humane doctor, which is good for the patient. Having one or two personal hobbies and interests and taking part in extra-curricular activities helps a lot in overall sense of fulfillment felt by the doctor. Any hobby is OK. It can be interest in art and literature or listening to or making music with instruments or singing or public speaking and not forgetting participation in sports activities. A well rounded person makes a better doctor certainly. But east or west, music is the best!

-

"The young doctor should look about early for an avocation, a pastime, that will take him away from patients, pills, and potions."
William Osler BMJ 1909;2:925-928.

-

<u>Music, O Music!</u>
Music, O Music, you touch and stir my soul,
Uplift my consciousness, and make me whole,
You make us forget ourselves,
Separateness evaporates, oneness alone prevails.
Music, O Music, O language of the soul!
Flowing from one to another soul,
You link all the souls-
'Oneness of all" that shows!
Music, O Music - a gift from the Mother Nature,
Who put music in the running brooks and in all creatures.
As also in soft breeze, sea waves, rain and thunderstorm,
So we and the happy Daffodils could swing, sway and dance.
Music, O Music, you're so natural to man-
In the hearty cry of the zesty newborn!
In the sweet chatter of a pretty infant,
Seed of music in all of us is forever implant.
Music, O Music, you're the element of prayer,
And the heart of a love song not so rare!
Music pervades just everything,
That is close to the heart of man!
Music, O Music, from ears you go straight to heart,
You make everyone sway in joy; shake and tap.
We all swing, swirl, jump and dance,
In such gay abundance as if in a trance!
Music, O Music, of flute and of drums,
Of Sitar, guitar, violin and other instruments!
Harmonious sounds make pleasant music,
Haunting melodies weave their magic.
Music, O music, beamed from my FM stereo-
One after another lovely song;
That keeps me happy as I walk or drive along,
God bless the DJ and may he live long!
Music, O Music - God bless those who make,
Happy, lively and soul-stirring music!

Be they Beethoven, Ravi Shankar or Yehudi Menuhin,
Jackson, Yanni, others, Khalid and Springsteen.
Music, O Music, could there be life without you?
Impossible, unthinkable, it's unimaginable too!
Life began with music, is sustained by it too,
Music is divine, the soul in me and you.
Music, O Music, life is ecstasy and picnic,
With love of music in it.
The breath of life is music,
There 'cannot' be life without it.
Music, O Music; O Music, O Music,
O Music, O Music; Music, O Music!

THE ART OF COMMUNICATION

Good communication is a necessary skill for doctors. A doctor
has not only to communicate with his or her patients but also has
to communicate effectively with his Professors, seniors, colleagues
and juniors. We are taught this through regular elicitation and
presentation of patient's case histories to the teachers; presenting
various topics in front of groups in seminar rooms and auditoriums
during our training period. We gain these practical skills and they
become part of our job skill set. Those of us who were initially
hesitant, they also pick up these skills.

Speak up!
From somewhere when I was a child, I read,
That 'Silence is Golden' and that got stuck!
But keeping mum, not talking became a handicap often,
I made no friends and was misunderstood often.
Although I remained a gentle, humble, harmless soul,
I was often labeled arrogant and self-centered bore.
I found no words to start an interesting conversation,
My handicap brought in me a feeling of desperation.
A sense of loneliness was fast growing up in me,
As I couldn't cheer anyone, no one ever cheered me.
Life became so boring, so dull and humdrum,

I badly needed a change and solve this conundrum.
I somehow wanted to break and shake away my shackles,
Get rid of my handicap, to profusely talk and chatter.
Dale Carnegie's, "How to win friends and influence people"
Liberated me as it taught me how to talk to and befriend people!
Living with and learning from great books and men,
I gradually transformed myself into an acceptable one.
Who liked to meet people, could talk to anyone,
Who took interest in others' lives and had with them fun!
Communication friends, is an art you aren't born with,
This skill can be learnt, acquired and mastered to the hilt.
You may learn music, drawing, acting, sculpting & others,
Art of communication has no parallel; you'll love it Sir!

P.S. The author read Dale Carnegie's book, 'How to win friends and influence people' quite early and revisited it many a times and found it useful. Dale Carnegie's book on Public Speaking is also quite useful.

PASSING THE FINAL MBBS/MD EXAMINATION

There are examinations at every stage of the course and the teachers test you at every step as to what have you learnt and grasped. You move forward to next year of the course if you have done well with the subjects assigned. And then comes the final examination after which you will be declared a doctor if you do well and pass. The exams are unending in the life of a doctor, even after becoming a doctor. Competitive exams for post graduate entrance and then exams for super specializations and exams and interviews for a job. How to manage an examination is also an art which a doctor must learn to perfection.

"With too many, unfortunately, working habits are not cultivated until the constraining dread of an approaching exam is felt, when the

hopeless attempt is made to cram the work of two years into a six month' session, with results only too evident to your examiners."

William Osler. Introductory Lecture on the opening of the Forty-fifth session of the Medical Faculty, McGill University, 1877. Canada Medical and Surgical Journal 1877;6(5):193-210

-

"Learn to see, learn to hear, learn to feel, learn to smell, and know that by practice alone can you become expert."

Thayer WS quotes Osler in "Osler the Teacher" Johns Hopkins Bulletin 1919:XXX;198

-

Win the MBBS/MD/MRCP Game!

Like every game has got its rules,
Its technique, style and its tools;
MD is different, but is a game all the same,
Most of its rules are laid out; it is a fair game.
You may play a game for pleasure and fun,
But you always like to win.
The boost that victory gives to your name,
Is so important in this career game!
This game is mostly played against professors of learning,
Who are on the other side and let the ball rolling.
With every question they ask the ball is put in your bin,
To give you a fair chance to hit and score and win.
Take a good social history in the long case,
Be systematic and thorough in every short case;
Think and answer well in the viva voce,
Stay cool throughout and you've won the race.
They are looking for some confidence,
Your accuracy and approach;
And if you scored a few clear goals,
A miss or two they would ignore.
In a short encounter of two hours,
They have to be forcefully convinced,
That you are capable and brilliant,

And can handle everything.
Once happy with your performance,
And convinced of your diligence;
They would stand up and usher you in,
And give you entrance to the Medical Fraternity of Fame!
-

-

P.S. The examinations are not always a pleasant experience. These are periods that bring stress. But stress can be overcome. This is how! The author once thought that he fared badly in the Anatomy practical exam and so was down hearted for a few hours. He then picked himself up and was back in enthusiasm for the afternoon session of the exam lifted up by remembering this quote:

"*Beeti ko bisaar ke, aage ki sudh le´*

Meaning: Forget the past; take now good care of the future.

At another time, the author once thought he wasted lot of time in gossips before his final MBBS examination and was getting anxious. Then what uplifted him to start work again with full energy was this quote, "Accept the worst!" What worst can happen? I will fail. OK, I accept it. After that I felt very light and ready to attack the preparation once again with full vigor and followed "Do your best"

-

NOW HAPPY TO BE A DOCTOR!

-

The young man is so happy that he has finally made it successfully to this prestigious and exclusive doctors club and is being honoured with the doctor's robes. In many colleges there is a robing ceremony day wherein they officially give you the doctor's white coat to put on. He is honoured and proud to be finally a member of this exclusive doctors' club for which he has been labouring and dreaming since many years. He now advises and invites all whom he can to join this exclusive club-The Doctors' Club.

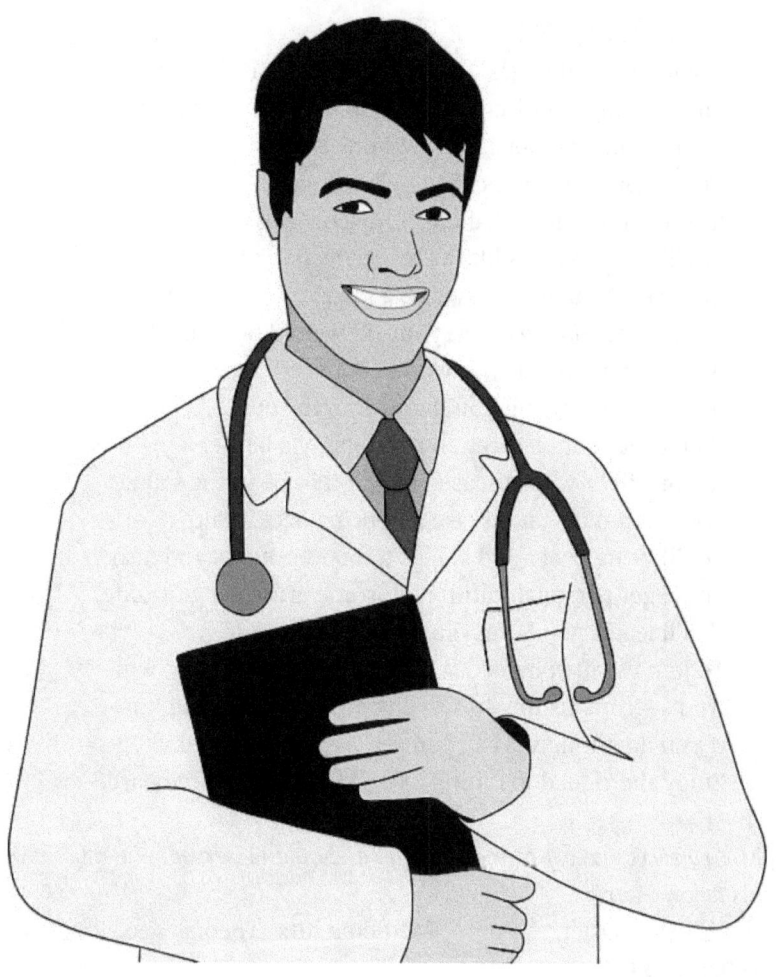

Finally! Happy to be a doctor!

-

"It helps a man immensely to be a bit of a hero-worshipper, and the stories of the lives of the masters of medicine do much to stimulate our ambition and rouse our sympathies."

William Osler: *Aequanimitas* 'Chauvanism in Medicine' 1914:288

-

The Doctors Club!
If you like challenges, love to explore the unknown,
Like a voyage of discovery and be like Sherlock Holmes?
Then come on youngsters join our club,
This exclusive one is called, "The Doctors Club."
It offers unlimited challenges, discoveries galore,
You'll pick up clues like a great detective of yore.
There's a stimulus every day, a puzzle at every turn,
If you love solving cases, your life would be fun.
Not a dull moment, you won't get bored,
A lot of excitement, you'll love it to the core.
You'll get your chances and win many a battle,
In your fight with disease, you'll often be in the saddle.
You'll often defeat disease and bring back health,
You'll bring cheer and smiles to many a home and hearth.
You'll get personal fulfillment, some grub and gratitude,
You'll lead a good life, you'll have an attitude.
To join us, all you need is curiosity and a desire to win,
And a strong feeling to serve your fellow kith and kin.
If you do strongly wish, you are welcome aboard,
Enjoy the ride; don't mind a few bumps while on board.

-

"To serve the art of medicine as it should be served, one must love his fellow man."

William Osler. Modern Medicine, Its Theory and Practice.' 1907;(1):34

CHAPTER TWO

A YOUNG DOCTOR IN TRAINING

A doctor is not just a bundle of information stored in his head as accumulated over the five years of classes in the medical school. A doctor is also a bundle of skills that he learns during the course of his practical training. He is also a bundle of empathy and sympathy towards his or her clients or patients. His knowledge and skills are to help the patients. After graduating, a doctor has to undergo mandatory minimum practical training of one year, called internship before he gets his certificate to practice.

The first thing a trainee has to master is how to conduct a patient interview. It has many components like history taking and physical examination. History taking itself has several components like Chief complaints, history of present illness, past history including past illnesses, drugs and surgeries, family history, personal and social history, history of travel etc. The Physical examination too has many components including general physical examination and systemic examination including cardiovascular, respiratory, gastrointestinal, genitourinary, neurological, bone and joint examinations etc.

"The whole art of medicine is in observation... but to educate the eye to see, the ear to hear and the finger to feel takes time, and to make a beginning, to start a man on the right path, is all that you can do."

William Osler. 'The Hospital as a College' Aequanimitas. 1914:332

-

"Get the patient in a good light. Use your five senses. We miss more by not seeing than we do by not knowing. Always examine the back. Observe, record, tabulate, communicate."

Abbott ME. of William Osler. The Pathological collections of the late Sir William Osler at McGill University. Bulletin of the International Association of Medical Museums 1926;IX: 185-199

-

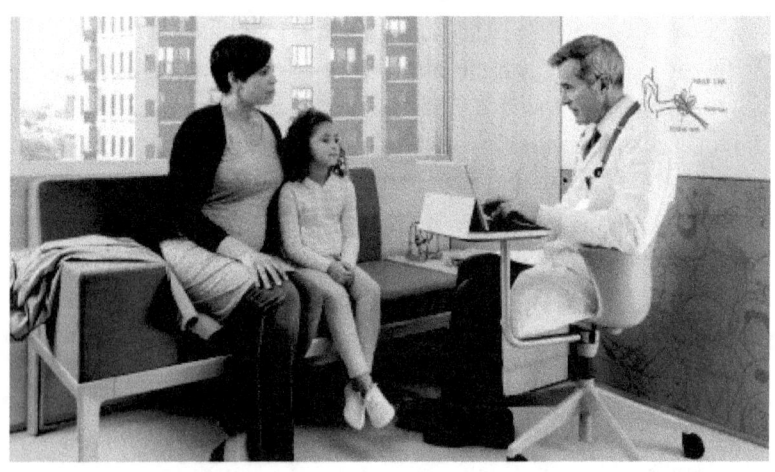

A doctor with a patient in the clinic!

-

Close Encounters of the Clinical Kind
While sitting in your clinic, waiting for the patient,
Talking to the nurse, you were getting for him impatient.
The reason for your existence is the patient you realise,
Your spirits are lifted, when he finally arrives.
Your welcome smile puts the patient at ease; ready for communication,
The nurse moves over, he is now the centre of your attention.

As the encounter begins, the clinician is all eyes and ears,
To watch facial expressions and demeanour; to what he says intently hear.
You listen to his story, with a sympathetic and open mind,
What ails, where hurts, what is not in order, as he finds.
You ask relevant questions, to fill the gaps in his story,
You don't forget his past, social, family or personal history!
Try to link, his present troubles, to his background,
Which organ system may be involved, try to make up your mind.
Don't miss any clues, O detective, of Sherlock Holmes' kind,
All observations create impressions on the astute clinician's mind.

From the chair, the scene then moves, to the examination couch,
The nurse at hand, curtains are drawn,
A careful, meticulous, unhurried, clinical examination is done,
To gather further evidence, about the organ system undone!
Be systematic; don't miss any step in the orderly examination,
For, the step you miss may hold the vital clue to your interpretation.
Please explain to him every step, of what all you do,
And don't you ever hurt him, by your word, expression or deed.
While the data gathering goes on let scientific thought proceed-
From the history, your observations and examination thus far-
You would have made up your mind, as to the system at fault,
Tell him gently your opinion; answer all his questions and doubts.

You suggest relevant investigations, to support your clinical diagnosis,
Then prescribe the medicine, to give him comfort and relief.
You may call him next time, to see test results and also know his progress,
But if it be serious or emergency, you refer and admit him to treat and assess.
Be honest in your assessment, sincere in communication,
Heal not only his body, but allay his fears and apprehensions,

In patient's relief and satisfaction, lies your gratification too,
If he leaves the clinic contented, he will come back to you!
This close clinical encounter may soon fade from your memory,
But impression you made on the patient, won't leave him easily.
He'll follow your instructions (hopefully), and do all you told him to,
And if he felt better it will please him (and you too) immensely.
Each close encounter, of this clinical kind,
Can be very vital (to you and the patient); do always keep in mind,
Your success in every case, builds up your confidence,
Ready for another encounter, yet another time!
In your success also lies the glory of clinical medicine,
And the success of William Osler, the teacher of bedside medicine.
If you follow these rules and play the game with such a plan,
Your sound 'clinical methods' become examples for all of medical clan.

-

"To study the phenomena of disease without books is to sail an uncharted sea, while to study books without patients is not to go to sea at all."

William Osler. Aequanimitas 'Books and Men' 1914:220

-

"Medicine is learned by the bedside and not in the classroom. Let not your concepts of the manifestations of disease come from words heard in the lecture room or read from the book. See, and then reason and compare and control. But see first. No two eyes see the same thing. No two mirrors give forth the same reflection. Let your word be your slave and not your master."

Thayer WS quotes Osler in "Osler the Teacher" Johns Hopkins Bulletin 1919:XXX;198

-

-

-

TAKING RESPONSIBILITY

A doctor in training is given gradually increasing levels and grades of responsibility. There is internship, then first second and third years of residency followed by senior residency etc. During the period of residency also studying and learning does not stop. He now studies about the patient he has seen in the ward or clinic, he looks up medical journals sometimes and he is learning new practical techniques while he is also preparing for higher studies and entrance examinations for furthering his qualifications. Gradually he becomes capable of taking decisions independently. Gradually he learns by imbibing from his seniors, how independent decisions are taken and what is the scientific process of decision making in patient care!

"The very first step towards success in any occupation is to become interested in it."

William Osler. Aequanimitas 'The Master word in Medicine' 1914:376

Responsibility!
Early in the profession I read somewhere,
"Responsibility Teaches", exhorted a Master.
For long I wondered how it might be so.
Then one day it became clear, behold and Lo!
During internship or residency and even after that,
The greater the responsibility you take upon yourself,
The greater you'll be learning, no doubt about that.
Shirk responsibility and you'll be a loser, it's a fact.
Some people are not eager or keen to learn,
Others avoid responsibility at every turn.
They must be disciplined and gently guided,
So that to them responsibility is imparted.
"Behave responsibly" is another good rule,
To guide us through the day's busy schedule!
Don't pass the buck or shrug off what looks tough,

Grapple with and solve problems to be leadership stuff.
Ability and freedom to respond is 'response-ability.'
How we respond to a stimulus is our distinct quality.
We are our masters in control, from now till eternity,
Being responsible remains our very own responsibility.

-

THE GROWING PAINS OF TRAINING

The years of internship and residency are not a cake walk. They are rather tough. Every third or fourth day you have a night duty where in you stay in the hospital during the whole night and anytime a new emergency patient arrives you have to attend to him or her and you have to take calls from the various wards of the hospital where the nurse will call you any time if she needs you for a patient's care. Many a night go totally without rest or sleep. When you start the next day, you can't just run to your home and rest. You have to first finish with the consultant the morning ward rounds and follow up the instructions and paper work after that, before you can call it a day. Many a time if there was a rain outside and the weather has changed the resident learns only after getting out of the hospital after 36 or more hours. In many residencies, for example cardiothoracic and neurosurgery, the length of duties could be even longer. With these long hours and duties, what happens to the young doctor besides his learning and training?

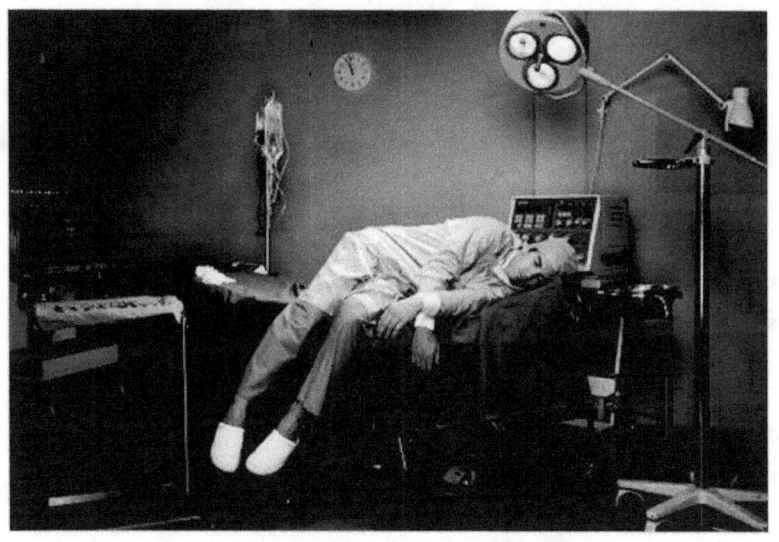

Over-worked, tired, exhausted!

-

Post Call Zombies!

With droopy eyelids, walking with us like a machine,
This young Doc is attending the rounds in a dream.
He has been 'On' since previous morning when bright,
He was on call, up and about, didn't sleep the whole night.
He now answers in monosyllables, understands little,
Miss-spells and miss-reads, is even slow to twitter.
His eyes are red, legs frail, brain very hot,
A little more and he will either shout or just drop.
This is not the first or the last time, that he knows is his fate,
It happens every third or fourth day and he can't escape.
It takes two days to recover; he can then see the next date,
He's wedded to the 'Duty Rota' for his career's sake.
Seniors won't help him for they have been through it all,
Since nobody helped them then, why now bother at all.
This is the eternal cycle through which all Docs must pass,

Like it or not, you have no choice, Alas!
Long hours prey on young Doc's health and take their toll,
They also make him thick skinned and insensitive to others call.
He may learn avoidance techniques, not respond to some calls,
Someone definitely suffers from this mismanagement of 'Calls.'
Now they've realized that our clients- the patients- do suffer,
If the doctor on call is not well-rested and doesn't appear
fresher!
If the nurses, pilots, factory workers have eight hour shifts,
Is the doctor super human to give quality in 36 hour shifts?
Now somehow though late, the wisdom has dawned, (1)
A shift of longer than 13 hours for doctors is banned. (2)
After the shift, for 11 hours they must rest and not work, (3)
The quality of care will improve as 56 hours a week, law works.
(4)
Young people have been deserting Medicine as a career for long,
They may now be brought back happily, they may sing a song.
We work for the good of the patient; we don't want any harm,
Let's have more doctors- dedicated to serve and charm!
-

References:

1. Rory Watson. On-call time in health centers must be seen as working time. BMJ 2000, Oct. 14, 321, 918.
2. NHS is not ready for a 48 hour working week. Rhona MacDonald. BMJ 2002, 25 May; 324: 1235.
3. Trusts are ill prepared for 58 hours a week for Junior Doctors. Katherine Burke. BMJ 2004, Feb 28; 328: 484.
4. Debashis Singh. Quarter of hospitals not ready to comply with working time directive. BMJ 2004, May 1; 328: 1034

-
-
-
-

RESEARCH –THE BEGINNINGS

This is also the time the young doctor is encouraged and is being trained in the methodology of doing research. How to frame a research question and follow it by gathering of data and drawing conclusions? How to do honest research and not fall prey to plagiarism? Few doctors develop interest in research depending upon their aptitude and needs of the job. The two primary ingredients of a research aptitude are Curiosity and then Creativity.

"To confess ignorance is often wiser than to beat about the bush with a hypothetical diagnosis."
William Osler. 'Counsels and ideals.' 1921:214

Curiosity
Knock and it shall be opened unto you,
That's true for every door.
Pass by, look the other way, or ignore,
It'll remain shut for you as ever before.
Ask and you shall be given,
Answers to the questions in your bubbly bosom!
Ask of yourself and that teacher Mother Nature,
Persistent alone find Nature's facts and secret features.
Do you ever wonder how this or that happens?
Then heed that wondering spirit before it dampens.
Don't suppress inquiry, let not the opportunity pass,
Exercise inquisitiveness, as does a little lass.
Curiosity is the key, to unlock every door,
Perseverance it'll take, to dislodge it some more.
Ask what, why and how, besides when, who and where,
Add imagination to intelligence, you'll get somewhere.
Let's not kill curiosity, as we grow old and older,
There's always more to know, but for those who are bolder.
Let's live life fully, accept or set no shallow limits,
Limitless is our nature, let's be true to our hearty spirit.

Curiosity is a vital tool, in the doctor's bag too,
A doctor is no good without this probing tool.
Questioning often leads to the cause of an affliction,
Treating the cause can earn some blessings and benediction.
-

Creativity!
The Spark of divinity that lies within you,
Carries the creativity of God enshrined in you.
There's an infinite store of creativity within us,
We just have to peep within and pop it out.
Man is most like God when he is creating,
All creations after man have been of man's making.
All that you need is to be passionately focused,
Your passion then creates the imagined object.
Scattered Sun's rays barely give some warmth,
But focused through a lens, burn a hole in a plank!
'Focus' is then what you need for being creative,
Scattered energy only dissipates that creativity.
What is it you want created; first have a clear mind,
Think about it in your awake and dreaming time.
Day and night you think only of that object,
A book, a machine, whatever shall materialize in fact.
Don't take much credit for any such creations,
You are His instrument; He is the Master of all creation.
Only recognize and hold that spark, that guides and goads you,
The rest will be automatic, stay focused, He'll lead you.
The 'Genie' is within, within each one of us,
Things do materialize through each one of us.
The degree of focus determines the degree of success,
Creativity is natural to us, for the divinity lives within us!
-

MAKING A DISCOVERY IS POSSIBLE!
The purpose of research is to find newer methods of diagnosing and treating the ailments that afflict man. When confronted by a challenging problem, a doctor must initiate research and dialogue

about the problem and make efforts and progress to discover new ideas, plans and solutions. All major training institutions train the doctor into research activities.

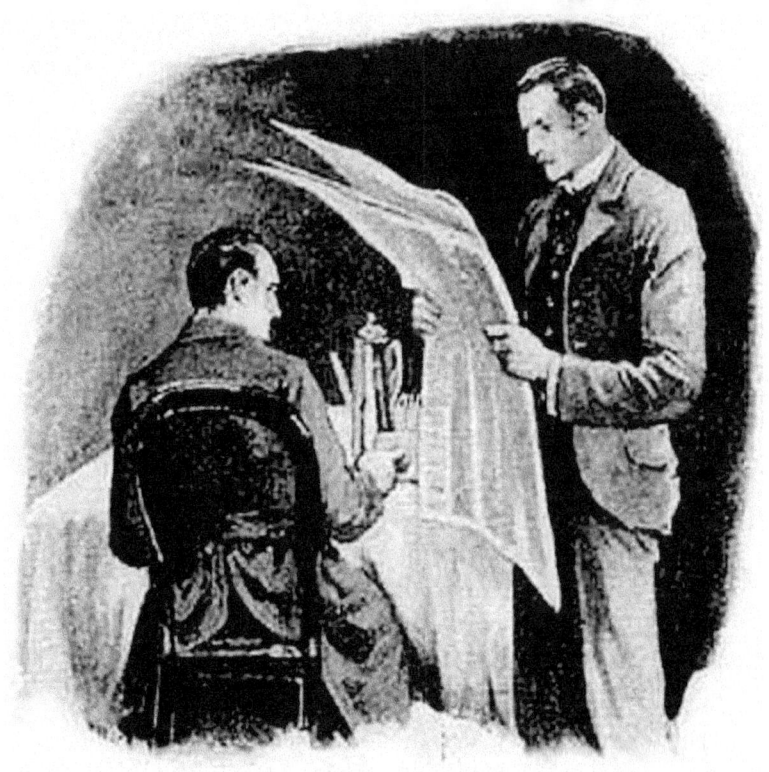

A Doctor has to be a problem solver and discoverer like Sherlock Holmes. Here Dr.Watson reading out the newpaper to Sherlock Holmes.

"One special advantage of the skeptical attitude of mind is that a man is never vexed to find that after all he has been in the wrong."
William Osler: The Treatment of Disease.Canada Lancet 1909;42:899-912.

-

"Medicine is a science of uncertainty and an art of probability."

William Osler

-

"Half of us are blind, few of us feel, and we are all deaf."
William Osler

-

"Learn to see, learn to hear, learn to feel, learn to smell, and know that by practice alone can you become expert."
Thayer WS quotes Osler in "Osler The Teacher" Johns Hopkins Bulletin 1919:XXX;198

-

<u>Discover, O man!</u>
What's this life, if you have not-
Discovered or invented something new?
What's the use, if you did not-
Push the evolution forward a step or two?
Service is essential, there is no doubt,
It ensures your survival, but that's it.
Human progress, if we were to bring about,
Discoveries unlimited are the path to it.
Be fired, motivated, inspired, O man!
Unravel, unearth, and unveil a new plan.
Mother Nature beckons a creative man or woman,
Explore, find or discover whatever you can!
Keep your eyes open, ears and other senses too,
Observe keenly, acutely, minutely, O you!
Draw inferences and put hypotheses forward,
Test them and conclude, and you've a discovery with you.
Sounds easy, so easy, yes you could do it,
Seeing is easy, but thinking, what about it?
What, why and how are the questions to ask,
Train your brain to strain to think answers to these.
Look for problems; put yourself in their very midst,
They're the stimulus, never evade, nor resist.
Look at them from every angle, ask relevant questions,
Persevere enough, discovery and invention will dawn upon you.

-

RESEARCH WRITING

Writing is an art which can be acquired. It is a necessary art for a researcher. When a research project is nearing completion with results ready for interpretation, the researcher needs to start writing about his research for communication to others through publication. There is a certain pattern in which the scientific research must be carried out and presented in the form of a presentation to an audience or sent to a journal for publication. Publivcation in a research journal itself is a process that takes time for the article to go through the Editor or sub editor, then sent for peer review to qulified referees and then back to the editor either approved or rejected or approved for publication following recommended corrections and improvements.

-

"There is no more difficult art to acquire than the art of observation, and for some men it is quite as difficult to record an observation in brief and plain language."

William Osler. Aequanimitas 'On the educational value of the Medical Society' 1914:357

-

"The greater the ignorance the greater the dogmatism"
William Osler

-

<u>On Writing a Scientific Paper</u>
"Publish or perish", they say and it's very true,
'To get published is no joke', I know is also true.
Writing a Scientific paper is hard at best,
To get it into a Scientific Journal is harder yet.
But you encounter some, who've written hundreds of them,
Not just written, but also successfully published them.
There must be a knack, an art, which could be acquired,
So that after learning it, we could do as well as required.
I learnt these secrets quite recently,
From a master who described them very succinctly (1).

Think and plan about your paper well in advance,
Get your message visible in the title at the first glance.
Follow IMRAD structure in all you write (2)-
Introduction: Any gaps in knowledge? Why you did it?
Methods: What you did and how you did it?
Results: What did you find? Tell in actual numbers,
Discussion: What's the meaning of your results?-
In themselves and in relation to the work of others!
If your paper follows all these rules,
And has a clear message which appears cool;
With proof supplied by the results you obtained,
Give a meaningful and catchy title; for it's your brain-child!
Before you send it, rewrite your article, remove distractions,
Better tell a colleague or two for criticism and corrections. (3)
It may save the trouble to the referee and the editor,
Who thus pleased will grab your neat and meaningful paper.
Writing alone begets better writing; for it is an art,
Each finished paper goes through four or five drafts.
Till the final product is precise and concise,
Without verbosity, rambling or grammatical vice!
If you can impress the referees and the editor -
Which is your aim and that you should monitor!
Then your success is guaranteed and ensured,
Your paper will see the light of print soon, rest assured!
If they send it back, don't lose heart, don't despair,
It may be for corrections and clarifications here and there.
And if they don't accept send to another journal by all means,
Persist and persevere till your important message is in print
seen.
"Have a message; will write a paper!"
Every scientist so thinks as he tries and digs deeper!
Every paper then becomes an important link,
In the long chain of human progress, so we think!
Amen! (Be it so).
-

REFERENCES

1. Whimster WF. Biomedical Research. How to plan, publish and present it. London: Springer-Verlag, 1996:264.
2. International Committee of Medical Journal Editors. Uniform requirements for manuscripts submitted to Biomedical Journals. JAMA 1993;269:2282-6.
3. Paton A. Write a paper. In: How to do it: 1. 2nd ed. British Medical Association: Oxford University Press, 1991:193-7.

-

-

-

GAINING WISDOM

Man does not live by bread alone. True. Man lives by wisdom. A man does not come with all the formulas for living. We need knowledge and wisdom which must be learnt and gradually picked up. One needs to make effort for this. Good people's company and good books are the sources from which right knowledge is imbibed. Wisdom is when knowledge is applied and experience gained. Wisdom is that which liberates and brings peace within and without. Practical wisdom can often be stated in a few words like one liners, two or four liners or small poems which can be learnt by heart. These short bits of wisdom become the quotes that we remember and live by in our daily lives and they often redeem us in our difficult times.

-

Quotations on the Wall*

We are born in ignorance, knowing nothing at all,
Blank looks, dependent for things big and small!
But potential energy lies latent, hidden in us all,
Parents and teachers kindle our flames as we crawl.
Slowly, steadily, we pick up valuable bits,
Through spoken and written pieces of wit.
Wisdom of ages put in one-line bits:
These quotations lead us, when we're at loss of our wits.

"Do to others as you wish to be done by."

"Look before you leap, think before you speak."

"No pains, no gains" "As much sugar so much sweet".

"Whatever you sow that only thou shall reap."

"Be good, do good" "Practice makes a man perfect."

"Work more, talk less" "A smile wins friends, at no cost."

"To err is human, to forgive divine" "Excess of everything is bad."

"Actions speak louder than words" "As the company, so is man"

Such quotations and a hundred more, strike our ears over and o'er,

We check them with our experience, make them our very own.

We then pass them onto next generations with our own notes,

Wisdom continues to live and grow; we all love witty 'Quotable Quotes!'

* Hurst J.W. Quotations on the wall. Ann Intern Med. 1999 Oct. 5; 131(7): 551-4

-

-

P.S. The author in his student days read and greatly appreciated the book of 'Essays by Emerson'. Ralph Waldo Emerson, an American philosopher has written essays on such subjects as, 'Compensation', 'Self Reliance', 'Spiritual Laws', 'Over Soul', 'Friendship' etc. Some of his words that greatly influenced and impressed me are: "Put your heart and soul in to the work that you will be judged by", "Pay for it and get it", "No pains, no gains" The essays are beautifully presented. The wisdom in his essays is great and practical. Here is a paragraph from the essay, 'Compensation':-

"POLARITY, or action and reaction, we meet in every part of nature; in darkness and light; in heat and cold; in the ebb and flow of waters; in male and female; in the inspiration and expiration of plants and animals; in the equation of quantity and quality in the fluids of the animal body; in the systole and diastole of the heart; in the undulations of fluids, and of sound; in the centrifugal and centripetal gravity; in electricity, galvanism, and chemical affinity.

Superinduce magnetism at one end of a needle, the opposite magnetism takes place at the other end. If the south attracts, the north repels. To empty here, you must condense there. An inevitable dualism bisects nature, so that each thing is a half, and suggests another thing to make it whole; as, spirit, matter; man, woman; odd, even; subjective, objective; in, out; upper, under; motion, rest; yea, nay."

-

Here is another paragraph from "Compensation"

"All things are double, one against another.—Tit for tat; an eye for an eye; a tooth for a tooth; blood for blood; measure for measure; love for love.—Give and it shall be given you.—He that watereth shall be watered himself.—What will you have? quoth God; pay for it and take it.—Nothing venture, nothing have.—Thou shalt be paid exactly for what thou hast done, no more, no less.—Who doth not work shall not eat.—Harm watch, harm catch.—Curses always recoil on the head of him who imprecates them.—If you put a chain around the neck of a slave, the other end fastens itself around your own.—Bad counsel confounds the adviser.—The Devil is an ass.

It is thus written, because it is thus in life. Our action is overmastered and characterized above our will by the law of nature. We aim at a petty end quite aside from the public good, but our act arranges itself by irresistible magnetism in a line with the poles of the world."

-

Here are a few lines from the essay, 'Self Reliance':

"Trust thyself: every heart vibrates to that iron string. Accept the place the divine providence has found for you, the society of your contemporaries, the connection of events."

-

"Whoso would be a man, must be a nonconformist."

-

"What I must do is all that concerns me, not what the people think."

-

"I suppose no man can violate his nature. All the sallies of his will are rounded in by the law of his being, as the inequalities of Andes and Himmaleh are insignificant in the curve of the sphere."

-

"Let a man then know his worth, and keep things under his feet. Let him not peep or steal, or skulk up and down with the air of a charity-boy, a bastard, or an interloper in the world which exists for him."

-

The essays can be found at this address: http://www.gutenberg.org/files/2944/2944-h/2944-h.htm

CHAPTER THREE

DOCTOR: NOW A FULL FLEDGED PROFESSIONAL

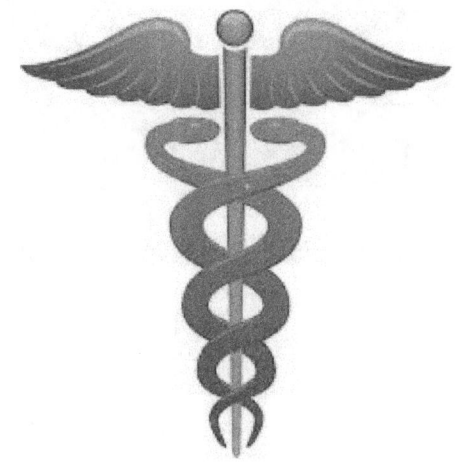

The Insignia of the Medical Profession.

By now, after years of training and work experience, the doctor has become reasonably well established in his profession and may have found some recognition in his circles. He might have seen hundreds of patients and treated them. He may be a member of some medical societies and groups.

A professional is one who professes or practices a profession or occupation or trade. The doctor now realizes his responsibilities and advantages that come with being a professional. Every act of his has to be measured and every step responsibly taken. By practising this way regularly, he becomes an expert in his field.

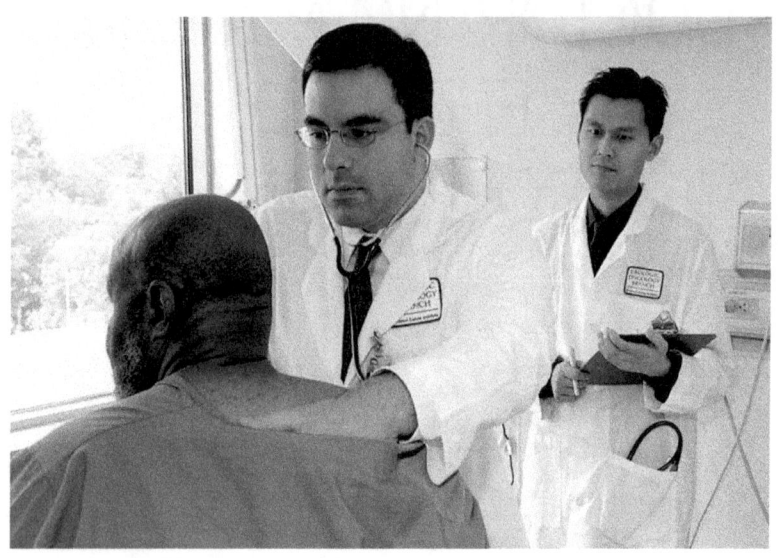

Doctor on ward rounds examining a patient.

-

"Every patient you see is a lesson in much more than the malady from which he suffers."
William Osler: Aequanimitas 'The Student Life' 1914:425.

-

<u>A Professional's Job</u>
Learn your trade well, baby
Learn your trade well!
It's going to pay you swell,
It's the source of your butter & bread.
If you know that you know
Your subject very well,

And 'can do' whatever
Need be done right and well;
You also often 'show' them,
That you know and can shine,
Let your confidence speak,
Through your 'confident smile'!
Whatever field you choose in life,
As your noble profession,
Your knowledge and enthusiasm to do,
Will take you to perfection;
You always try and stay ahead,
Show your worth by solid actions,
You will reach where you want to be,
And get a job satisfaction.
People are everywhere people,
If you watch them intently,
They are often easy to impress,
You only act confident naturally;
If you come forward and talk,
Show them figures and your facts,
Or raise important questions,
You may then hold them in your grasp.
This is what a job is all about,
We gain experience by and by,
Knowledge and experience sure make,
Experts with authority!
It is experts that the world needs,
And experts we shall be,
If we fulfil the needs of the world,
We shall be fulfilled too.
So, learn your trade well, baby,
Learn your trade well,
'Show' them what you've done,
And achieved so well;
If 'you' don't proclaim yourself,

Others can only guess,
They under-estimate a quiet man,
So come forward and tell.
Baby, come forward to tell!

-

LEARNING IS A CONTINUOUS PROCESS IN A DOCTOR'S LIFE

-

O I learend so much; O I am tired of learning; these kind of thoughts, a doctor never entertains because he can't afford to. In the life of a doctor learning is a continuous and long term and almost an endless journey, often exciting. One has to take it very positively and enthusiastically. If that attitude is there, there is no stopping the progress in a doctor's life.

-

"If the license to practise meant the completion of his education how sad it would be for the practitioner, how distressing to his patients! More clearly than other the physician should illustrate the truth of Plato's saying that education is a life-long process."
William Osler. 'An address on The Importance of Post Graduate Study' Lancet. 1900;156(4011):73-75

-

"For the general practitioner a well-used library is one of the few correctives of the premature senility which is so apt to take him."
William Osler. Aequanimitas 'Books and Men' 1914:221

-

"The higher education so much needed today is not given in the school, is not to be bought in the market place, but it has to be wrought out in each one of us for himself; it is the silent influence of character on character."
William Osler

-

Learning all the time!
Knowledge is now expanding at such a fast pace,
To keep up-to-date is not unlike a race.

What was known as true when you entered medical school -
If you repeat it while leaving, you may be called a fool.
Even if you know today what all is there to know,
By tomorrow new studies make a mockery of all you know.
So, it's important to keep one's eyes and ears always open,
Let the old practices pass and imbibe the new trends that open.
These are the days of practicing "Evidence Based Medicine":
Of Randomized Controlled Trials (RCTs); Meta-analyses based medicine.

You can't base your practice just on a Professor or a book's advice,

You must learn to educate yourself of what's latest in your science.

You must also know what we don't know for sure,
Ask relevant questions, look for or set up a RCT and explore.
All new treatments must pass through this rigorous route,
You accept them only if p is < 0.001; that's significance absolute!
Learning must never be over, we must learn all the time*,
It's a sign of life; it keeps us in tune with our times.
A doctor's life is being on a cycle; you stay upright if you pedal,
You fall into oblivion if you stop to learn and fail to pedal.
But all said and done, learning is nothing if not fun,
If you take it as a burden, it's your problem- you'll be undone.
Let's labor to learn and also labor to spread what we learn,
A lit candle lights another, that's how our luminous world runs!
*It's good to talk: Thoughts for new medical students at a new medical school.
Richard Smith, Editor BMJ. BMJ 2003, 20 December; 327: 1430-1433.

-

WHAT ARE THE EXPECTATIONS FROM THE DOCTORS?

-

Although the profession gives us respect in the society but there are so many expectations that as professionals we must fulfill. It has been experienced that if you do right in hundred instances and fail in one, the hundred are totally and immediately forgotten and on this one instance a doctor is taken to task. A doctor quite often feels he is on tenterhooks all the time. There are great expectations and demands from the society from him.

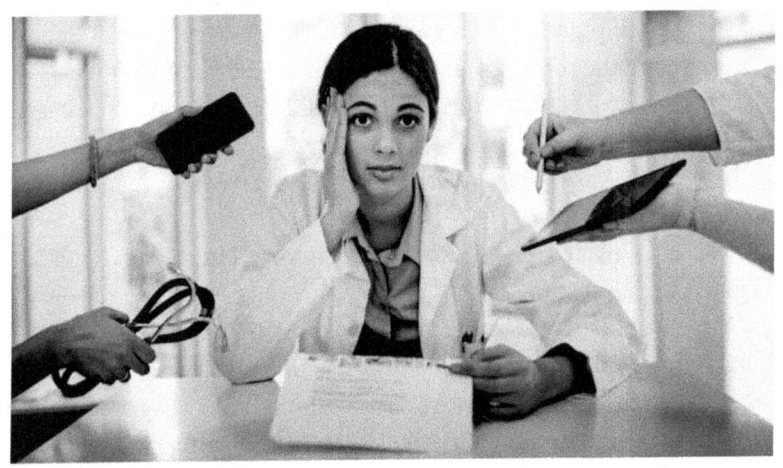

Doctor, please sign here; please attend a patient's call; doctor, there is a call from the ICU(Intensive Care Unit)!

-

"Work is the open sesame of every portal, the great equalizer in the world, the true philosopher's stone which transmutes all the base metal of humanity into gold."

William Osler. Aequanimitas 'The Master-word in Medicine' 1914:373

-

"The practice of medicine is an art, not a trade; a calling, not a business; a calling in which your heart will be exercised equally with your head. Often the best part of your work will have nothing to do with potions and powders, but with the exercise of an influence of the strong upon the weak, of the righteous upon the wicked, of the wise upon the foolish."

William Osler. Aequanimitas 'The Master-word in Medicine' 1914:386

-

<u>Great Expectations, Great Demands!</u>
One of the oldest professions in the man's world on earth,
Promoter of health and life; enemy of disease and death,
Physician in the society is in great demand,
From the doctor the public has great expectations, great demands!
All doctors are bound by the Hippocratic Oath,
To keep interests of the patient upper most.
They call it therefore, a noble profession,
Doing good to all - what a great expectation, great demand!
He must serve with a smile, be ever helpful and kind,
Solve all problems, of body, soul and mind,
He should restore health and allay also fears,
He is not God; yet, great expectations, great demands!
He must keep all self-interest in abeyance,
Must be always available, charge only a pittance?
Must live simple; be sober, wise and also bland,
From his noble profession, great expectations, great demands!
To make a good doctor, takes such a long time,
Five years of education, several years of training time,
The grinding that a doctor in the making undergoes,
Is truly tough; but is his profession's great expectation, great demand!
A doctor must work on, day and night
Often over the assigned 56 to 72 hours a week,
Yet he must be alert, awake and right in mind,
He is not super-human, yet it's a great expectation, great demand!
A doctor mustn't smoke or drink or drug,
Set an example, be a picture of health instead,
Stay cool and calm; satisfy patient's needs, demands,

Live happily even under stress; it's a great expectation, great demand!

Medical knowledge is growing, at a rapid pace,

Merely to keep up-to-date, you have to race,

He must know the latest, on finger-tips of his hand,

From this hard working genius, great expectations, great demands!

Continuous professional development or CPD is a must,

Continuing medical education or CME must go on,

Both are necessary just to stay in the profession,

Recertification every 7 years! That's a great expectation, great demand!

You be sincere, do good and right all your life,

But make some mistake they'll hold you tight.

Authorities or patients may take you to court,

Stress and tension, part of life, of great expectations, great demands!

But if you love this ancient profession of yore,

If service to mankind is your goal and forte,

Such highly motivated and dedicated doctors find,

Great satisfaction, great rewards; despite great expectations, great demands!

-

HOW DO DOCTORS FEEL PRACTICING THEIR PROFESSION?

-

The medical profession creates mixed feelings in the mind of doctors. It is tiring, demanding of time and energy and yet it is rewarding in term of social stature and a reasonable lifestyle and a sense of personal satisfaction. During our everyday practice we face unlikely situations and challenges. We face challenges of reaching a correct diagnosis, treating the patient well physically and psychologically. Besides we also see lot of pain and suffering. That also affects us.

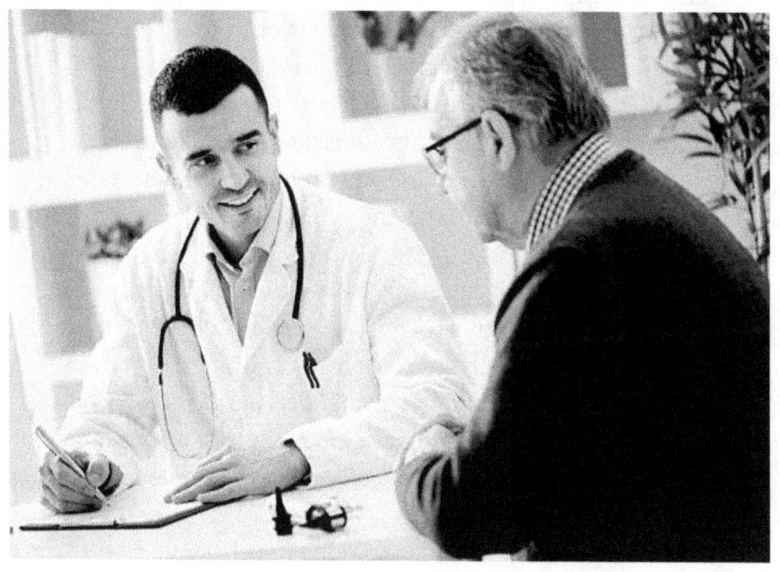

A pleasant doctor keenly listening and reassuring a patient.

-

"Courage and cheerfulness will not only carry you over the rough places of life, but will enable you to bring comfort and help to the weak-hearted and will console you in the sad hours when, like Uncle Toby, you have "to whistle, that you may not weep."

William Osler. Aequanimitas 'The Master-word in Medicine' 1914:386

-

"Things cannot always go your way. Learn to accept in silence the minor aggravations, cultivate the gift of taciturnity and consume your own smoke with an extra draught of hard work, so that those about you may not be annoyed with the dust and soot of your complaint."

William Osler. Aequanimitas 'The Master-word in Medicine' 1914:385

-

-

Our (Doctors') Lives

Doctors see so much misery all their lives,
At such close quarters, through days and nights.
So much pain and suffering; the departing of human lives,
It's strange how lasting sorrow, doesn't grip our lives.
A sense of scientific aloofness and philosophical detachment,
Urgency of attending the next challenge keeps us from attachment.
The observed human suffering, we keep as an external event,
If we internalised all this sorrow, we couldn't survive an instant.
We must be protecting ourselves in several ways,
To stay alive, healthy and happy and partake of life's plays!
We sympathise and empathise, with a fellow's sorrow and pain,
But get energised and activated to relieve someone's hurt or pain.
The sense of achievement in the relief of others' unease,
The sense of mastery in the cure of symptom and disease,
The challenge of bringing disease and sickness to an end,
Is enough to keep us kicking and go beyond any narrow ends!
The rewards are not small; they too keep us going,
We share the joy and happiness, of a relieved and cured fellow being,
Joy of a baby being born; a child getting well, the relief of loving parents,
We celebrate and toast the health, of each health restored patient.
The sense of gratitude shown and the feeling of 'God' we are given,
Is so overwhelming, encouraging, uplifting and humbling even!
We then redouble our efforts, to master our techniques,
To conquer disease and to give relief!
Our lives are busy, there is no doubt,
There is often little time, for family and pleasure routes.
But surely we lead purposeful, meaningful and useful lives,
In God's creation, we couldn't have asked for any better lives!

-

P.S. At this point, the author remembers a famous poem called, 'If' written by Rudyard Kipling, possibly advising his son on the value of Self confidence.

'If'

If you can keep your head when all about you
Are losing theirs and blaming it on you,
If you can trust yourself when all men doubt you,
But make allowance for their doubting too;
If you can wait and not be tired by waiting,
Or being lied about, don't deal in lies,
Or being hated, don't give way to hating,
And yet don't look too good, nor talk too wise:
If you can dream—and not make dreams your master;
If you can think—and not make thoughts your aim;
If you can meet with Triumph and Disaster
And treat those two impostors just the same;
If you can bear to hear the truth you've spoken
Twisted by knaves to make a trap for fools,
Or watch the things you gave your life to, broken,
And stoop and build 'em up with worn-out tools:
If you can make one heap of all your winnings
And risk it on one turn of pitch-and-toss,
And lose, and start again at your beginnings
And never breathe a word about your loss;
If you can force your heart and nerve and sinew
To serve your turn long after they are gone,
And so hold on when there is nothing in you
Except the Will which says to them: 'Hold on!'
If you can talk with crowds and keep your virtue,
Or walk with Kings—nor lose the common touch,
If neither foes nor loving friends can hurt you,
If all men count with you, but none too much;
If you can fill the unforgiving minute
With sixty seconds' worth of distance run,

Yours is the Earth and everything that's in it,
And—which is more—you'll be a Man, my son!
Source: *A Choice of Kipling's Verse* (1943)
-

DOCTOR PATIENT RELATIONSHIP
-

One of the most important subject in a doctors life is the kind of relationship a doctor should have with his patients. There is a Hippocratic Oath that we doctors take and that is our guiding principle in dealing with the patients, our clients.

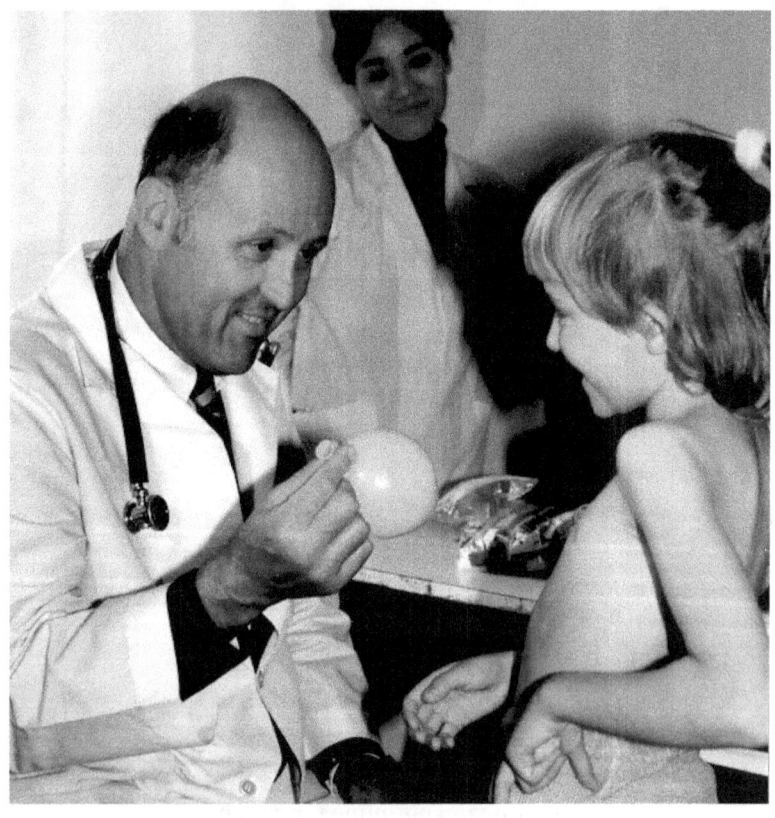

Doctor patient relationship- a Pediatrician with a happy child!

-

"The good physician treats the disease; the great physician treats the patient who has the disease."
William Osler

-

"The first duties of the physician is to educate the masses not to take medicine."
William Osler

-

<u>The doctor patient relationship</u>
The doctor sat in one seat and the patient sat the opposite,
There was a distance between them of about four feet.
There was no physical connection between the two,
And yet somehow they seemed connected too.
There was the apparent client-provider connection,
That is the usual part of any social transaction!
There was an element of faith and goodwill connection,
That is essential for this kind of interaction!
But there was yet some more subtle and spiritual connection,
Being invisible, though vital, it's not the accepted convention.
This one is not an ordinary but inseparable connection,
So obvious but missed, this is the heart to heart connection.
We are so closely connected a doctor has to make an effort to stay aloof,
If we were indeed different we won't be taught to stay objective, affect-proof.
We all pretend we are different for practical reasons of transaction,
Deep inside we all know we have a deeper, much deeper connection.

-

-

P.S. On Doctor patient relationship, the author came across a poem which expresses another dilemma that doctors face often. It is so difficult to treat a patient when he is your close relative or a family member. It is often recommended that doctors don't treat themselves or their family members. The reason is that emotions come in between and can destroy the neutrality of the doctor patient interaction; may also hamper the relationship because of expectations and complaints. This dilemma is expressed nicely by Dr Dannie.

"X-ray" by Dr. Dannie Abse. A Welsh poet, editor, playwright and novelist, Dr.Dannie Abse(1923-2014) was a physician who practiced in London. In this poem "X-ray", Dr Dannie reflects on the age-old problem of treating one's own family, here his mother.

"Some prowl on sea-beds, some hurtle to a star,
And, mother, some obsessed turn over every
stone or open graves to let the light in.
There are men who would open anything.
Harvey, the circulation of blood, and
Freud, the circulation of our dreams,
Pried honorably and honored are like all
explorers. Men who would open men.
And those others, mother, with diseases
like great streets named after them:
Addison, Parkinson, Hodgkin—physicians
who would arrive fast and first on any
sour death-bed scene.
I am their slowcoach colleague, half afraid,
incurious. As a boy, it was so; you know
how my small hand never teased to
pieces an alarm clock or flensed a
perished mouse.
And this larger hand is the same. It
stretches now out from a white sleeve to
hold up, mother, your X-ray to the
glowing screen.
My eyes look but don't want to; I still
don't want to know."

-

The poem finds mention in the book " Medicine: A treasury of Art and Literature" and can also be found at this URL where the original source of the poem is also given.

https://www.poetryfoundation.org/poetrymagazine/poems/34137/x-ray-56d21793976b8

PATIENT FIRST

A doctor always keeps the interest of the patient first. He not only treats his physical ailment but he also deals with him very humanely to unburden him of his worries. There may be worries about reaching the doctor, fees of the doctor, waiting time in the clinic, buying the medicines, being regular in taking the medicine etc etc. A doctor listens to all problems of the patient very sympathetically and tries his best to help him. He can't do everything for the patient himself, he advocates the patient's case in front of others to get solutions to his patient's problems.

"Care more particularly for the individual patient than for the especial features of the disease."

William Osler, Address to the students of the Albany Medical College.Albany Medical Annals. 1899;20:307-309

Doctor: an advocate too!
He comes to you with a health complaint,
Listen to a patient's story real well.
Make up your discriminating mind,
What is wrong and what's not well.
He comes to you and surrenders,
Hoping his secrets you won't tell¶*.
He puts his trust and faith in you*,
Do everything to see that he gets well¶.
If it's a simple problem,
You solve it yourself*.
If it requires a specialist referral,

You *advocate* his case with skill and deft.
You may be called as an expert witness,
In the land's courts of law!
There you *advocate* on his behalf,
His medical case without a flaw!
If occupation is the reason,
For his sundry health problems;
Advocate to his employer a change in his work,
So in safe and healthy environs he may work.
Always *advocate* the welfare of the patient,
Advocacy is part of a doctor's job! (1)
To *advocate* the health and welfare of Society at large¶,
A doctor again is neatly cut for the job.
"Doctors against War and Nuclear Weapons,"
"Doctors for Universal Healthcare and Immunizations!"
"Doctors against Tobacco, alcohol and Drugs,"
Doctors' voice is heard; speak up, don't shrug.
So if you happen to be a doctor,
Your profession demands you to be an *advocate* too (2).
Hone your skills of public speaking,
Speak for individual's health and society's welfare too (3).
'Profession' from Latin, means 'Speaking Forth', (4)
So come on doctor, get up now and start speaking forth.
*Devotion to service, profession of values*and *advocacy,*
This *Medical Professionalism*(4) leads to social adequacy!
References:

1. The doctor's role in advocacy: Editorial. Richard Horton. The Lancet; Feb.9, 2002, Vol.359, 458.
2. Medical professionalism in the new millennium: a physicians' charter. Medical Professionalism Project. The Lancet; Feb.9, 2002, Vol.359, 520-22.
3. Medical professionalism in the new millennium: a physicians' charter. Medical Professionalism Project. Ann Intern Med 2002; 136: 243-46.

4. Medical Professionalism in Society: Sounding Board. New England Journal of Medicine. Nov.18, 1999; 341: 21; 1612-1615.

Symbols: ¶ **The three fundamental principles**for medical profession: Principle of primacy of patients' welfare, Principle of patients' autonomy, Principle of social justice.

* **The Ten Commitments**and professional responsibilities of doctors and the medical profession : Commitment to professional competence, Commitment to honesty with patients, Commitment to patients' confidentiality, Commitment to maintaining appropriate relationships with patients, Commitment to improving quality of care, Commitment to improving access to care, Commitment to a just distribution of finite resources, Commitment to scientific knowledge, Commitment to maintaining trust by managing conflicts of interest, Commitment to professional responsibilities.

-

ABERRATION OF THE SACRED RULE

-

Patient first is the rule which is always followed by all doctors. But in these days of commercialization of medicine, many patients feel that doctors have become more commercial and looking after their own interests first rather than of their patients. Patients express it in many ways, like the doctor charges an exorbitant fees, the doctor orders un-necessary investigations, the doctor advises un-necessary surgery etc and all this to make more money for himself, his hospital or for his institution just to make his own place secure there. These allegations may all be partially true, but what do the doctors say on this? Doctors complain that people give money to their plumber or electrician without grumbling but when it comes to paying a doctor they feel the doctor should treat them for free, being a noble person.

-

"Perhaps no sin so easily besets us as a sense of self-satisfied superiority to others."

William Osler: *Aequanimitas* 'Chauvanism in Medicine'
1914:284

-

*"By far the most dangerous foe we have to fight is apathy –
indifference from whatever cause, not from a lack of knowledge, but
from carelessness, from absorption in other pursuits, from a contempt
bred of self satisfaction."*
William Osler: *Aequanimitas* 'Unity. Peace and Concord'
1914:457

-

Betrayal of trust!
When the patient felt hot and not a clue he got,
He surrendered, "Help me doctor, you're my God."
That's a profound, deep-felt, faith sublime,
Doctors do respect it; keep patients' interests prime.
But at times one sees, with surprise and distress,
Some use his helplessness, for their greed and success.
And often in such a shameless and a blatant manner,
Their compromise with conscience seems total and final.
True, the doctors are after all human beings,
With stomachs to feed, cravings and some needs.
But when their survival depends on patients' pockets,
The risk of exploiting their patrons is great for their profits.
When business and commerce enter doctors' hearts,
Kindness, sympathy and uprightness do simply depart.
Their thinking, outlook and paradigms change a lot,
Money is the centrepiece of the new values they've got.
They order unnecessary investigations and procedures,
Justify them to the ignorant and entrapped customers.
Devious methods are employed to fleece innocent folks,
It's strange, how some of us can stoop so low; us blokes!
And here follows the reasoning and advice from seniors:
"If a horse were to start loving the grass,
It would soon perish, it won't last.
So hike your fees and take your referral cuts,

Procedures bring money, order some part cut."
"And if we don't order, the use of our machines,
How shall we take out our costs, O you novice trainee?
Let them call it cheating, fleecing or betrayal of faith,
Be thick-skinned; play tricks of trade for survival's sake."
Save me O Lord, from such crooked thoughts and ways,
Make me a doctor, but only as your servant always.
Give me enough for me and my family's needs,
Let me live contented within my legitimate means.
Let me not compare with rich nor have a trader's dreams,
Keep me away from greed; please don't let me be mean!
Let me be true to my profession, not spoil its name,
Let me serve thee, in thy beings, O Lord, Amen!
-

P.S. The author one day in the library, while going through the two books mentioned below came across a poem that represented the views of public on doctors, expressed beautifully.

"Doctors" by Anne Sexton, Pulitzer Prize winner 1967(Live or Die)

They work with herbs and Penicillin.
They work with gentleness and scalpel.
They dig out the cancer, close an incision,
And say a prayer, to the poverty of the skin.
They are not Gods, though they would like
to be;
They are only human, trying to fix a human.
Many humans die. They die like the tender
berries in November
But all along the doctors remember:
First do no harm.
They would kiss if it would heal.
It would not heal.
If the doctors cure, then the sun sees it.
If the doctors kill, then the earth hides it.
The doctors should fear arrogance more

than cardiac arrest.

If they are too proud and some are, then
they leave home on horseback and God
returns them on foot.

-

MEDICINE- A TREASURY OF ART AND LITERATURE
Ann G. Carmichael & Richard M. Ratzan. 375 pages, 8.5" x 11",
Full-Color, English, 2016.
Originally published by Hugh Lauter Levin Associates, Inc., 1991.
https://global-help.org/products/medicine-a-treasury-of-art-literature/

MEDICINE-AN ILLUSTRATED HISTORY
Albert S. Lyons & R. Joseph Petrucelli, II. 618 pages, 8.5" x 11",
Full-Color, English, 2016.
Originally published by Abradale Press, 1987.
https://global-help.org/products/medicine-an-illustrated-history/

The above two books are a great resource for those interested in
the history of medicine and art and literature associated with it. The
books can be downloaded for free in pdf format

-

DOCTOR: PRACTICE WHAT YOU PREACH
A doctor is a part of the society and the social milieu in which he
develops. He also may pick up some social and personal evils on the
way. His body like others may get addicted to certain substances,
the most common of which is cigarette smoking. He also is a victim
of addiction and can't get rid of it. When he advises his patients
against smoking, it does not cut much ice with them, for they know
the doctor himself is smoking. Smoking smells; patient can smell.

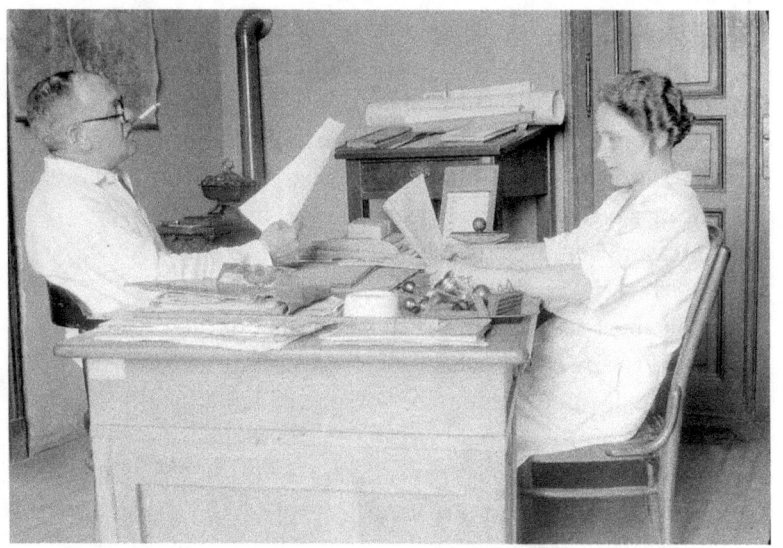

The Puffing Doctors!

-

"Some of us are congenitally unhappy during the early hours, but the young man who feels on awakening that life is a burden or a bore, has been neglecting his machine, driving it too hard, stoking the engine too much or not cleaning out the ashes and clinkers. Or he has been too much with The Lady Nicotine, or fooling with Bacchus or worst of all with the younger Aphrodite- all 'messengers of strong prevailment in unhardened youth!"

William Osler in 'A way of life'

-

<u>The Puffing Docs!</u>
When I tell a patient with bronchitis cough,
That smoking is bad and it should be stopped,
He laughs at me and answers back, "Sir, if
Smoking were really that bad for health,
Why so many of your tribe, the Docs would puff?"

That shatters my confidence to convince the patient,
I am forced to keep quiet at that moment.
But strangely, when I tell a patient of heart attack pain,
That smoking is the cause and it should be stopped,
The answer is always, "I would never ever smoke again".
On follow up I do see, that most indeed have quit for good!
Puffing a cigarette, blowing smoke rings into skies,
Is pleasure and fun but only until when?
The pain attached to the act is felt and clearly seen,
As the most severe pain which nearly shatters all dreams.
I wonder why only a catastrophe is required,
To wake us out of the slumber of feigned ignorance,
Simply to notice the bold writing on the wall,
"The evidence is strong that smoking is the cause of it all".
In this matter, doctors, are no different from laymen,
The urge and compulsion to go and smoke, is stronger than,
The force of factual knowledge they may have,
Devoid of a painful experience, this force fails to force.
In a corner of the hospital, away from public gaze,
There is a room where the Docs may smoke,
They have several pretexts to puff and fume,
For concentration, to relieve tension, or constipation,
Or for indigestion and to stay slim!
All nice reasons, but all cooked up,
For, don't they pass motion who never got hooked up?
The danger they know is very real,
But heart attacks they feel happen only to other people.
The real culprit, Sir, is Lady Nicotine,
Its grip on the brain cells is strong and keen,
The dependence is both physical and psychological,
So no more than 3 % smokers per annum can quit1.
Within eight seconds of the first puff2,
Nicotine reaches the blood and the brain cells,
The cells get excited and ask for more,
Little wonder then, that cigarettes are,

The most addicting Products known!1
The best way to quit, friends, is not to begin,
For fun or adventure or just to stay slim3,
Prevention here, is better than cure,
Educating kids can work for sure.
Ban tobacco advertisements or ban public place smoke,
These partial measures, would only partly work,
Stop tobacco cultivation, stop its imports,
We may lose tobacco revenues, but save in health care costs,
We save lives, health, happiness and environment the most.

-

REFERENCES
1. Henningfield JE. Nicotine medications for smoking
cessation. N Engl J Med 1995;333:1196-1203.
2. Sylvis GL, Perry CL. Understanding and deterring
tobacco use among adolescents. Pediatr Clin North Am
1987;34:363-77.
3. Califano JA, Jr. The worng way to stay slim [Editorial].
N Engl J Med 1995;333:1214-6.

-

WHEN PATIENT VISITS A DOCTOR IN THE HOSPITAL

A patient when he comes to visit a doctor in the hospital, he is
not very happy about it because he knows he is not visiting a picnic
spot. He has problems that bring him to the hospital. He has many
apprehensions in his mind about how he will be dealt with, what
will the doctor do to him, how much time it will waste, what will be
the advise he would be given and how much it all would cost? With
all his worries he lands in the hospital clinic and what does he go
through?

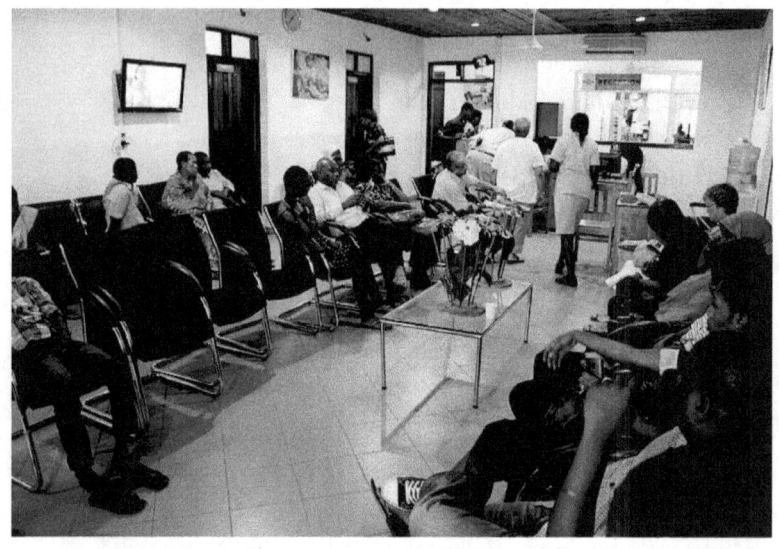

Patient's patience gets tested in the waiting lounge of the
Doctor's clinic.

*"It has been said that 'in patience ye shall win your souls,' and what
is this patience but an equanimity which enables you to rise superior to
the trials of life?"*
William Osler, *Aequanimitas*. 'Aequanimitas' 1904-4
-

A Patient's patience!
I know what it is to 'be patient',
For I was recently a hospital patient!
They test your patience all throughout,
From entry to the moment you are out.
In the hospital, a doctor is the big boss-
Can't see him without an appointment pass!
Such a long wait before the offered date,
I felt small and humble not important or great.
Was in real bad need so I kept the appointment,
Reached before time only to my disappointment!

My file wasn't ready; the clerk wasn't there,
"There are many before you, you may sit down Sir."
I had left my work halfway in my office,
My boss allowed but wanted me back in a trice.
And here I was asked to relax and kill time,
Boss came to my mind on every clock chime.
An hour later, we witnessed a furor in the crowd,
Might be busy elsewhere, now the doctor had arrived!
Everyone had their eyes glued to the doctor's door,
What a big relief, to see number one ushered in-door.
Number two, three, four, and the calling came to a halt,
From the back door had entered a member of the staff!
After a full twenty minutes number five was called,
Everyone was angry but could only murmur to oneself.
I was restless, couldn't sit, started pacing the floor,
Who entered or exited, my eyes riveted on "the door."
My pacing then came to a sudden standstill,
The doctor quietly went wherever he willed.
Upset but helpless a patient couldn't do a thing,
Thankfully the 'doc' was back perhaps after a drink.
I hoped and prayed no more staff should fall sick,
So the doctor may see us in order and relieve us quick.
For a moment I wished I had known some hospital staff,
I would have been treated as a V.I.P and be quickly off.
"Oh God my B.P is going up I can't take it anymore,"
Then I heard the sweet sound of my name from "the door".
I collected and calmed myself, put on an artificial smile,
'Good morning doc', pretending everything was fine.
No complaints about delays and the disorderliness,
I rather got on with the story of my own illness.
I was exposed and examined, touched here and there,
My calm and patience were tested as I lay there 'bare'.
I dressed up and waited, for the doctor's verdict,
But it wasn't final, "Come after tests in another week."
"Ö God, my job would go tell me what should I do?"

"Son, go to the lab, stand in another queue!"
"What God, do you care or don't you care about me?"
"Patience son, patience; when you are healthy or ill"
I listened to my God stood in every other queue,
Was back in the clinic in exactly a week too!
Going through this ordeal has made me 'very patient',
Visit to the doctor makes you much more than 'a patient'.
-

PATIENT NEEDS ADMISSION

Sometime the patient can't be treated on the out-patient basis. His condition demands it and he is too sick but perhaps does not realize the seriousness of his condition or is too apprehensive. The doctor then has to use all his art of convincing to get the patient on the hospital bed for his own good, thus allaying his apprehensions about what may happen.

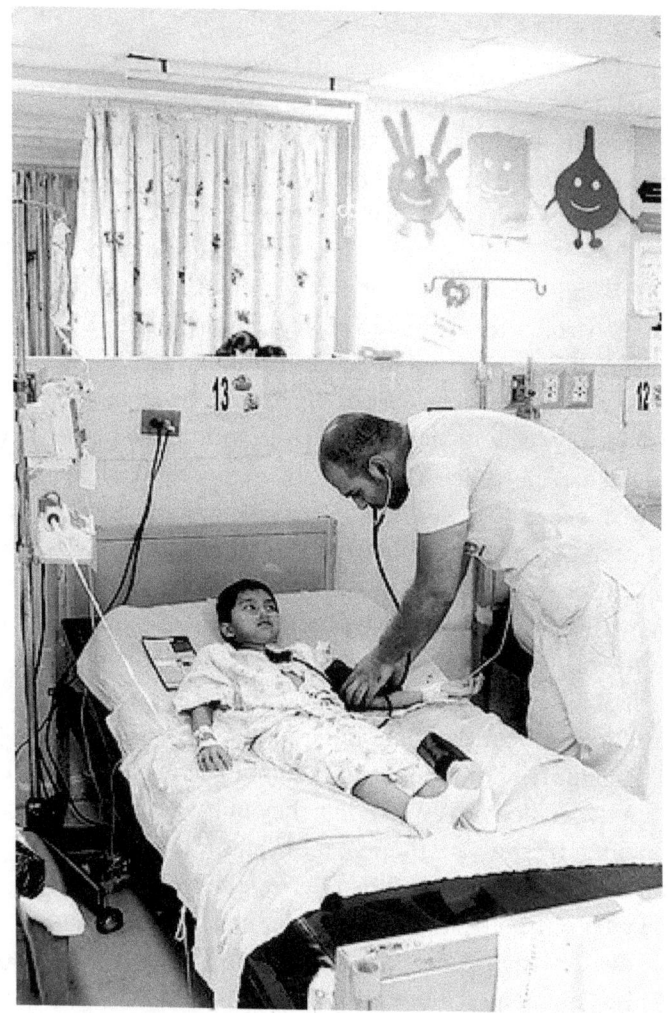

Checking blood pressure of a child on the hospital bed!

-

"It is much more important to know what sort of a patient has a disease than what sort of a disease a patient has."
William Osler

-

The Hospital Bed

The thing we dread is the hospital bed,
Though well-cushioned and with a fine linen spread;
Its comfortable looks give no peace; create fear instead,
A hospital bed is a hospital bed, a thing we dread.
A modern hospital bed, is not an ordinary bed,
It's all steel, a mini-machine, and a gadget in fact.
Pull the railings or elevate it and depress it at every third,
You may roll it from place to place or lock it instead.
This machine costs no less than a fortune to get,
The daily maintenance cost to the hospital is no less.
Perpetually in short supply, this contraption, the hospital bed,
Creates no cheer, doesn't eliminate fear, repels instead.
Why this fear, why this dread, from the humble hospital bed?
Whose intentions are only to give comfort and rest!
"O God! Save me, please save me from the hospital bed"
"Why this prayer, what have I done?" asked the noble bed.
It's the fear of sickness, fear of ill-health; fear of unknown,
Inevitable surrender to doctors of more or less renown!
Besides this the real pain of innumerable needle pricks and pins,
And a hundred limitations on freedom; you're at staff's whims.
From the endless investigations, they put you through,
You often feel you are their goat or a guinea pig!
Junior and the senior staff handle you the way they please,
You are now theirs; as you happen to be just a 'bed number six.'
The disruption of personal and social life, and the long delays,
The loss of independence and uncertainty of what happen may?
All these are no small reasons, to fear the hospital bed,
So much so, that for some, it's a constant nightmare ahead.
A bed is a bed, is a bed after all; depends on how you assess,
A bed at home and hotel denotes health and happiness.
A hospital bed is bad news, means vulnerability and sickness,
And varying amounts of anxiety, tension, depression and stress!
But dear friends, life is ever in a state of perpetual motion,

Health like everything else is not an ever-lasting condition.

So, when your train on sickness station stops;

And nothing gives you comfort, relief, solace or props-

You may then, find all these on the hospital bed,

And then, please don't stay away in dread,

From this otherwise feared but well-meaning hospital bed,

To cross and pass from sickness station back to vigour and health!

The greatest benefactor of sick mankind is a hospital bed!

Look at positives, don't dwell on negatives; teaches us the hospital bed!

The number of patients sent home happy and well,

Speaks volumes on the goodness of 'our hospital bed'!

-

LISTEN TO ME DOCTOR!

-

Not to the doctor directly, but amongst themselves and when with their relatives many patients complain that the doctor did not listen to them carefully. Rarely they will tell the doctor about this.

They complain especially if the medicine or the advice given to them did not work and he did not feel better. The doctor has then to be very patient himself and listen to their complaints with an open heart and a helping attitude.

-

"Keep a looking glass in your own heart, and the more carefully you scan your own frailties, the more tender you are for those of your fellow creatures."

Homan E quoting Sir William Osler: Teacher and bibliophile. JAMA 1969;210:2223-5

-

"Listen to your patient, he is telling you the diagnosis".

William Osler

-

-

-

<u>Can't feel my pain?</u>
<u>Please listen to me doctor!</u>
"Poor listeners", yes physicians are poor listeners,
People with chronic pain see physicians as poor listeners.*
The Institute of Medicine committee on pain has so found,
This 'sadly' they felt and reported is the reality on ground. **
Most physicians have poor education and training in pain management,
A quarter of primary care physicians 'feel unprepared' in its management!*
In their regular clinics physicians are busy with so many sundry complaints,
In their ignorance of pain management, they ignore patient's pleas on pain.
Physicians' unscientific knowledge and attitudes towards pain relief-
Are the major impediments to patient's relief and worsen his grief!
They have fear of giving stronger medicine for patient's chronic pain,
Their fear of causing addiction is irrelevant in relief of cancer pain.
Why pain relief should be limited to only pain specialists?
When pain is so common, shouldn't it be known well by generalists?
Why pain education is not included in medical curricula?
Why patients have to suffer for our lop-sided curricula?
A patient comes to a doctor for his symptom relief,
If a physician can't do that it damages patient's faith and belief.
No use of any good intentions if a doctor is not well trained:
Pain relief is basic medicine in which all of us should be trained.
How can the doctor educate the patient about his pain?
He himself is so uneducated about the cause and relief of pain.
The Institute of Medicine has offered sixteen recommendations,
**

They include students' and clinicians' prompt pain care education.

*Pizzo PA, Clark NM. Alleviating Suffering 101—Pain Relief. New England Journal of Medicine. Perspective. 2012, Jan 19; 366, No.3, 197-99.

** Institute of Medicine, Relieving pain in America: a blueprint for transforming prevention, care, education, and research. Washington, DC: The National Academies Press, 2011.

-

FAITH IN THE DOCTOR

-

Not all patients complain about the doctor. Many get well and sing praises of the doctor too. Most patients have faith in their doctor. Faith heals as they say. Perhaps it does. Perhaps it does not. But positivity versus negativity clearly are different in their overall outcome of any action. Positivity maintains peace of mind and this may generate the release of good hormones called endorphins from the body and that may then help healing.

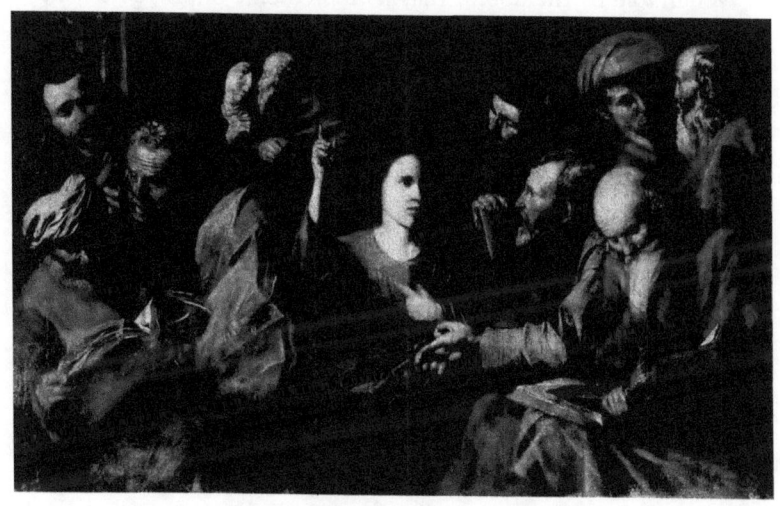

Christ among the doctors! A painting by Jusepe de Ribera(1591-1652)

-

"One of the first essentials in securing a good-natured equanimity is not to expect too much of the people amongst whom you dwell."
William Osler
"The greater the ignorance the greater the dogmatism"
William Osler

-

<u>Faith first, Life next</u>
Sitting on the edge of the hospital bed, leaning forward,
He* was blue and breathless, breathing hard.
He complained of nothing, as the doctor asked him, how he was,
He said with a smile, 'Al-hamdulillah' or 'Praise be to the Lord'.
In his faith he had lived and survived all his life,
When disease struck him, death was near; nay rife!
He didn't abandon his faith, or start complaining to God,
Situation was grim but he said, thanks to God.
When told by the doctor that with medicine improve he will,
He only said, ' Inshaallah' or 'only if God so wills.'
He knew, nothing could move without the will of God,
He kept his faith; first in health and now on his sick bed.
Such enduring, abiding faith is not hard to find,
It keeps them contented, happy and satisfied in mind.
Endless complaining about life and what it gives or brings,
Is not part of their belief, training or upbringing!
Accept whatever comes, as it comes from Him,
That is what the faithful have been brought up in.
Keep strong your faith through thick and thin,
Into the heaven of eternal peace you'll be taken in.
* A real patient in Oman.

-

-

-

-

WHAT IS DOCTOR'S FAITH? JUST BE GOOD, DO GOOD!

-

Whereas a patient has faith in the doctor's healing power and through that his getting better, his faith that the doctor is good and will do good is also deep seated. A doctor is trained to be good and do good. The dictum for the doctor is, 'Above all do no harm.' Doctor's personal satisfaction lies in just this, that he was good to his patient and did his best for him. The ultimate healing and cure is really beyond him also. There are many other unknown factors that play a role in the overall healing process. But the doctor must do his part sincerely and to the best of his knowledge and capacity and very honestly.

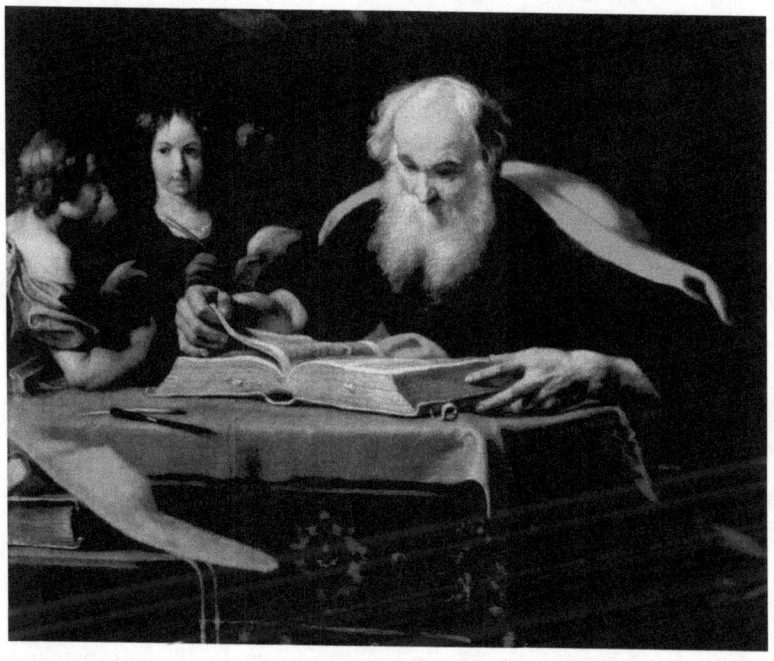

The Four Doctors of the Western Church! A painting by Gerard Seghers(1591-1651)

-

-

-

<u>My goodness!</u>
All our lives, we keep wondering where is God?
We seldom realize in goodness itself is God.
God is goodness, and goodness is God,
God is good, everything good is therefore God.
When you're in real trouble, hoping for some help,
A Good Samaritan arrives and saves you with his act.
Don't you inside feel God Himself arrived on the scene,
He listened to your prayers and sent the Good Samaritan in.
Wherever you see goodness, know God is there,
If you have some goodness, God is surely in there
Wow! God is there hidden in each of us, you know,
While we look for Him in heavens He is smiling at us now!
Do good to your friend to make him feel about God,
Do good to your enemy and make him think of God.
Be good, do good, sounds so good, for so good is God,
See goodness all around you and in goodness God.

-

-

P.S The author is influenced by the high ideals of 'Vasudha-aiv-kutumbukam' meaning, the whole world is one family; and words like, 'Maitrah' and 'karuna' and 'nirvair sarva bhuteshu' and 'Advaishta sarva bhutanam'. Maitrah means friendship, karuna means kindness, nirvair sarva bhuteshu means no enemity towards all beings and advaishta sarva bhutanam means no jealousy or envy towards all beings. The author has lived in Arab countries and the USA and found that these principles are universal and applicable and applied everywhere. That is the beauty of being human.

That is how doctors are and need to remain. That transforms into doctors love for humanity shown practically as kindness and compassion and keeping patient's interest above everything else.

CHAPTER FOUR

DOCTOR AS AN OBSERVER OF LIFE

A doctor is trained to be a keen observer and express his observation in a lucid way. He observes various phenomena of life and death and some of them at very close quarters. He witnesses people dying of and suffering from addictions; he sees patients who are suffering due to poverty and nobody seems to care for them; he sees young people getting addicted to drugs and losing their youth to drugs and alcohol; he observes the elderly in the society and the neglect they suffer at the hands of the society as well as their near and dear ones. All these observations make an impact on his life.

"The value of experience is not in seeing much, but in seeing wisely."
William Osler

POVERTY AND HEALTH

Medicine these days seems to be out of reach of the poor man and his family. There all kinds of quacks sitting in the streets and giving qualified practitioners a run for their money. These quacks are the only recourse for the poor people in the society. Howsoever we may dislike the quacks for their quackery; they are there for a reason. They are the saviours of the poorest of the poor in the social strata.

Poverty is the enemy of good health in many ways, but strangely a doctor has no means to take care of this social malady. He has to live with it and help the needy as much as he can. He can not go in to the causes of poverty and ignorance and change the society at large.

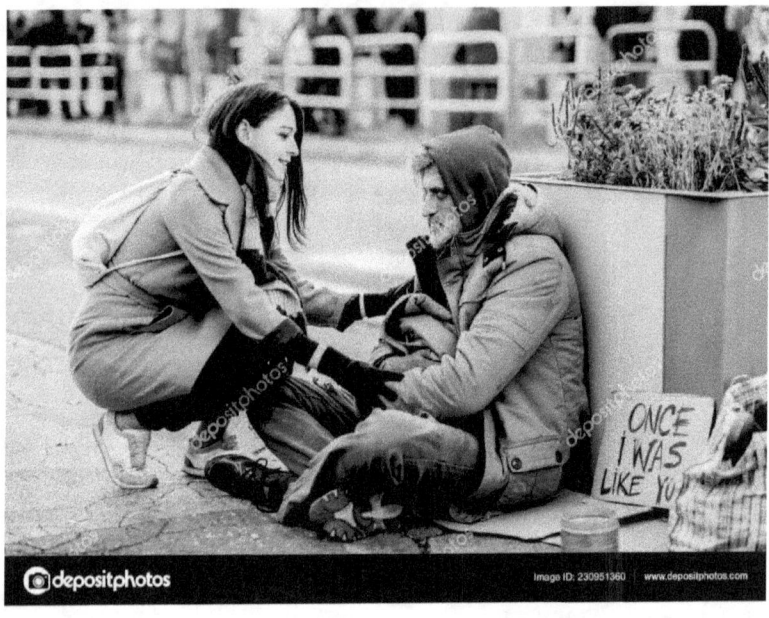

Someone cares for a Poor man!

Poor man's Health: Who Cares?
He slept by the roadside, this homeless man,
Few clothes, no possessions, had this man
Exposed to the cold, heat, dust and dangers,
Among society's garbage, lived this poor man.
There was another, with a meagre shelter,
He would beg or engage in menial labour.
Six members of a family to support he had,
Neglected by society, outcast he felt, this poor dad.
Some people thus live on society's fringes,
Starvation is close and real, on daily bread life hinges,

Making both ends meet, is a struggle indeed,
"Not fit to survive", in Darwin's evolution creed.
'Poverty is a curse', so the saying goes,
It debases the body, mind and soul,
Poor often succumb to the rigors of existence,
Poor nutrition, poor health and a mere subsistence!
For people living in the city's ghettos and slums,
Poverty is seldom the only problem,
Illiteracy, ignorance and superstition abound,
Apathy of rulers makes their problems compound.
Overcrowding in the slum-dwellings, their stuffy indoors,
Exposure to the nature's raw elements, outdoors,
Health facilities don't reach, the poorest of the poor,
No wonder, certain ailments are endemic and endure.
Lack of resources, personal hygiene and sanitation,
Lack of strength, a voice or enough education,
Are reasons why infections and malnutrition prevail!
That cut down the life-span, of our society's frail.
We blame the poor for all their ills,
Look the other way, to get away from feelings of guilt.
Who indeed is responsible for their fate?
Society's cruel rules or its rich and great?
'Survival of the Fittest', a rule of the jungle may be,
What'll be a civilised human society, if that were true?
Human mind sure is, not just an animal mind,
Kindness, and compassion in abundance, you may find.
If all of us who 'have', helped those who 'have-not',
Poverty's effects could be cut, if not halved at a trot.
We won't feel guilty of accumulating wealth,
If we shared some of it, with society's poor instead!
If all rich and able followed this prescription,
And didn't hesitate from service or conscription!
The world will become a much better place to live,
Men will not only hoard, but full of love, also share and give!
Amen ! Be it so!

OLD AGE AND CARE ISSUES

Another social malady the doctor faces is that as the people get older, say beyond the earning age of 60-65 years, they not only develop more and more diseases and disturbances in body's systems due to body's degeneration, they also feel societal and familial neglect in so many ways. That is painful for the doctor to see and hear every day. Lately however, governments have woken up to realize this neglect and have instituted a number of facilities for their Senior Citizens and are also spread of awareness among families to take nice care of their elderly.

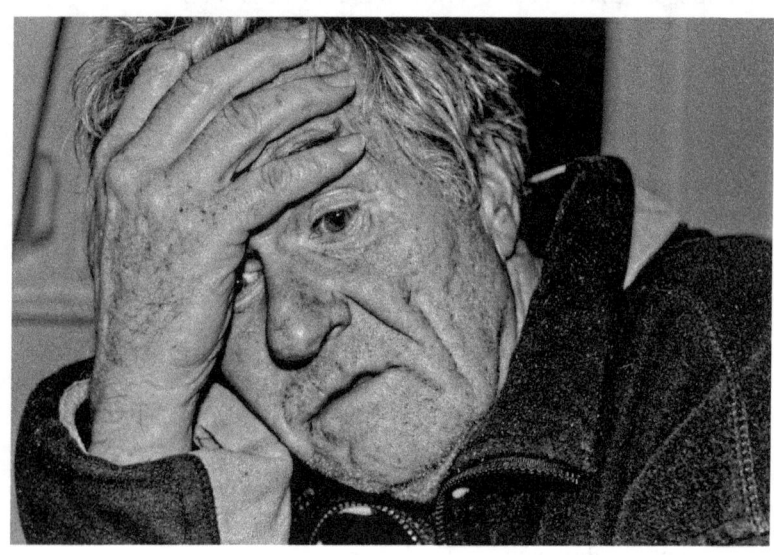

Worries of old age!

<u>Our elderly: who cares?</u>
Everyone likes the rising Sun, the bright Sunshine of dawn,
For we all love, energy, activity, strength and brawn.
But alas! Every dawn ends up in dusk -
The power, energy, action wane yet there's great glow at dusk!

When you are born it's your rise, it's your dawn,
You are the magic, and a wonder, for your loving dad & mom.
You can't feed nor bathe yourself, you can't walk or converse
You can only piss and cry, yet you are the centre of their Universe!
They feed, clean, dress and protect you, be it day or night,
Not for days or months but from infancy till you are bright.
They lead and guide you step by step, until you are safe on your own,
Theirs, my dears, is a labour of love; it's not for a later gain.
Time never stops, and the years fly by, we like it or not;
Age catches up with them, their systems begin to rust and rot.
Teeth fall and hands shake, knees pain and their legs are frail,
Walking and feeding are hard; and God forbid if memory fails!
Immobility, Instability, Incontinence and Intellectual failure,
Are the dreaded four 'I's, that all elderly fear.
When they are helpless and dependent in their twilight years,
Your carers then need caring for!
Their call for help and tender loving care often falls on deaf ears,
Doesn't go far!
Those who helped you walk and talk, call you now,
But for you survival is hard; you've no time for their care somehow!
No income, no resource, they aren't useful any more,
Wisdom may be there, but who listens? Who cares?
A burden, a nuisance, a headache, a sore,
These old ones, you can't take on, no longer, no more.
You wish, you hope, if someone else could care,
And do the job which, you know, is truly yours,
To look after your old ones in their disabled years -
'The elderly should belong to the Community', you're sure.
Geriatric Hospitals and Elderly Homes are a blessing & a boon,
For those elderly who can't find love or care at home in their afternoon.
But the stay at these places is against their wishes,

The trauma of neglect and rejection weighs heavy on their souls!
Neglect is the malady, the elderly suffer from,
Not by strangers, but by their near, dear & loved ones!
Those loved ones for whom they shed their sweat and tears,
Are busy with their own cares; won't shed for them any tears.
Loneliness, cruel loneliness; nurses can't cure loneliness,
No Kith or Kin; no grandchildren to see or to talk,
No smiles, no cheers, no respect; no hustle or bustle,
All hope is lost, melancholy takes a firm grasp.
Blessed are the elderly, who, in their dusk years,
Are cared for by their loved ones, living with their dears,
So they feel wanted, loved, respected; content and pleased,
Till one day, the Sun sets finally, and sets their souls free!

-

THE CHALLENGE OF CARING FOR ELDERLY WITH ALZHEIMER'S DISEASE

Caring for elderly who are developing dementia and Alzheimer's disease can be specially challenging for the relatives in the family. The family of such patients needs full support from the health institutions and doctors. The Carers here need to be supported fully psychologically as they themselves get prone to develop stress, depression, sleeplessness, exhaustion and a sense of getting fed up and a tendency to give up.

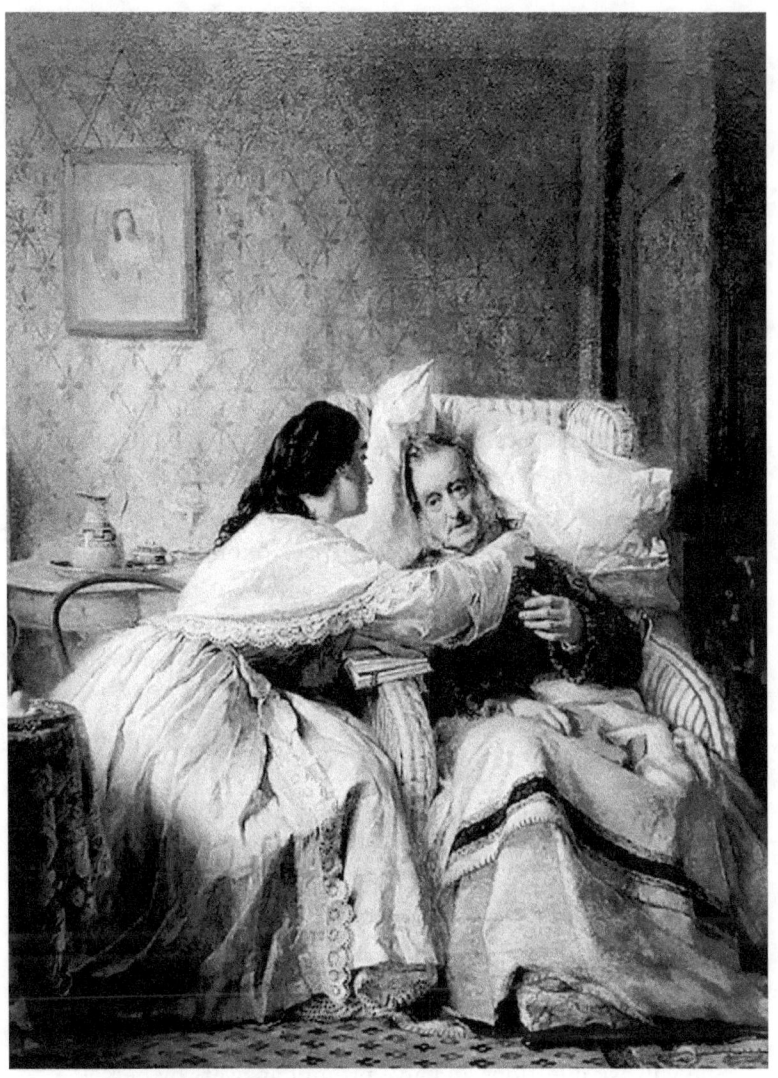

Woman's Mission, Comfort of Old Age! A painting by George Elgar Hicks(1824-1914).The Tate, London.

-
-

-

<u>Watch your elderly!</u>
She was always at the door wanting to go out,
She knew they had come and they called her out.
Thus for house keys, she was always on the lookout,
'Who locked the door? Give the keys, I must go out.'
She tried to open the door with whatever she found,
Be it the car keys, the scissors, even a tablet round.
She would stand at the window asking them for keys,
'Get me the keys, do give me the keys.'
Finding the main door closed one day,
She thought there must be another way.
She entered the bathroom, was confronted by the mirror,
She returned saying, 'A grey haired old lady is blocking my way!'
She always tried to cook for her long gone Dad,
She wanted to make dough to make bread for her Dad.
She made the dough from the washing machine soap one day,
We kept the 'Tide' box on top of the fridge from that day.
Ask her to brush her teeth:' I have already done that!'
Please take a bath: "Well, why again, why never you?"
Please flush the toilet: 'Why should I, you used it, why don't you?'
Please change the clothes: 'What is wrong, they are clean.'
Please come, eat your food, 'No, I am not the least hungry!'
Please go sleep on your bed: 'No, I'll sleep here on the sofa!'
Let's go for a walk: 'No, I don't want to go, you go!'
To any suggestion she was always in the mode called, 'No!'
For hours on end she will talk to herself,
She'll talk to her sisters and others just by herself.
She will ask questions and give prompt answers by herself.
Noisy and often loud, she kept busy all by herself.
She would often laugh and giggle with them,
She would sometimes cry for the death of someone.
When in a 'self-talking attack', she was hard to distract,
She won't sleep herself, nor let us rest!

Her son came to see her from a far of land,
After two days she told him, 'Why you are wasting your time?'
"Go, do your work or your wife will throw you out this time."
Poor fellow felt bad when he saw what he saw of his Mom this time.
We went to the doctor and told him her story,
He diagnosed her Alzheimer's; which is some old people's story.(1)
He gave some medicines to keep her calm and for sleep,
But the course he said is unremitting till the final sleep!

-

1. Hebert LE, Scherr PA, Bienias JL, Bennett DA, Evans DA (August 2003). "Alzheimer disease in the US population: prevalence estimates using the 2000 census". *Arch. Neurol.* **60**(8): 1119–22. 'Alzheimer prevalence was estimated to be 1.6% in the year 2000 both overall and in the 65–74 age group, with the rate increasing to 19% in the 75–84 group and to 42% in the greater than 84 group.'

-

CHILDREN ARE PRECIOUS

-

Children are the direct face of God. Sweet, innocent, dependent; they need to be taken care of very well by the parents, family and society at large. They are the future of a society and the nation of tomorrow. Children are indeed precious and divine, rich or poor alike. Quite often society forgets to recognize that they too have rights which must be respected. Children's psychology and needs must be understood and supported by the healthcare teams and society in general.

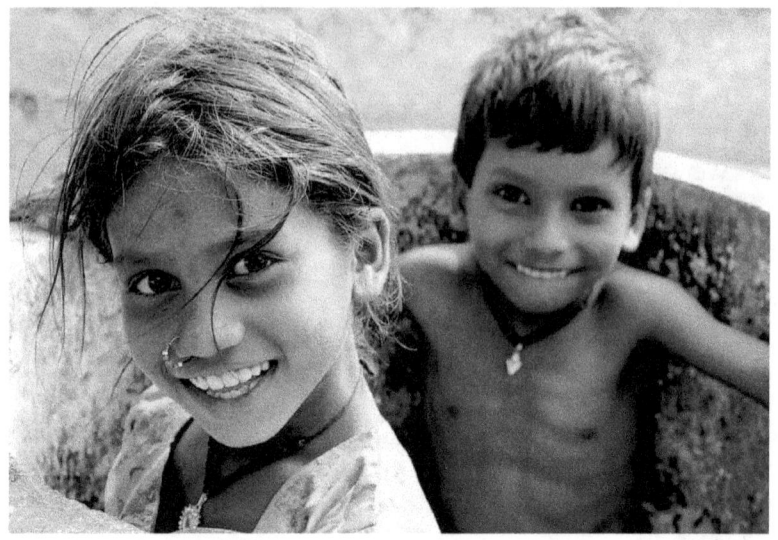

Children's rights must be recognised, respected and ensured!

The Children's Rights

Children are children just like flowers are flowers,
Rich man's or poor man's kids are all flowers!
Flowers will charm you; you maybe whoever,
Rich and poor kids charm you wherever, whenever!
Kids need the right environs to blossom and to flower,
Or the bud shrivels, doesn't bloom into a flower.
We must take care no bud ever shrinks before it flowers,
Society must ensure that the poor man's kids too flower!
One day, when your car stopped at a street red-light,
You saw kids begging; were you moved by that sight?
Have you seen kids scavenging for food in a waste dump?
Did that scene not give you quite a few goose bumps?
These kids belong to slums; they're the poor man's chums,
No sanitation, no school, no education; bare huts, no fun.
Here poverty, illiteracy, malnutrition, disease go hand in hand,

Come on, here you will find a bud that needs a helping hand!
Every child that is born on earth must have these four rights:
Right to survival: good nutritious food &healthcare is the first right.

Right to development: to quality education, care and recreation,
Right to protection: from harm, neglect, abuse and exploitation.
The last of the four rights is not the least, it is no concession,
Right to participation: to freedom of thought and expression!
They don't need our lip-sympathy; they do need some action,
When their rights are subverted we must stand up, rise in action!
Bravo! Three cheers for all kids!

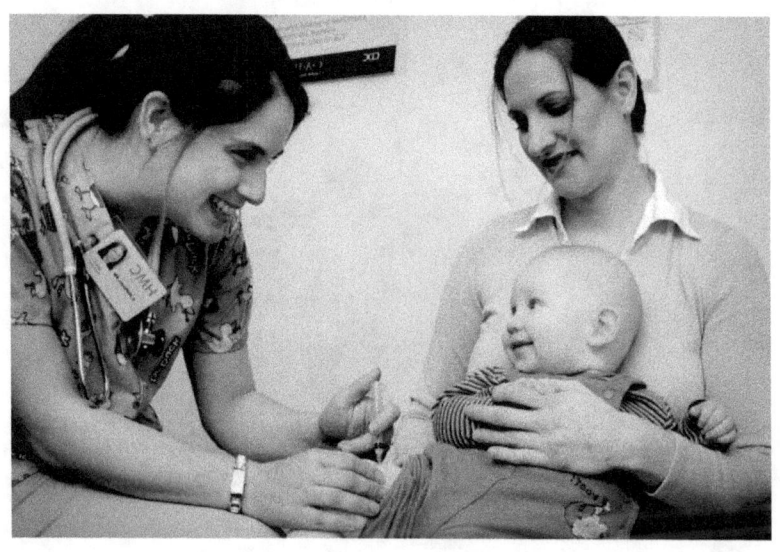

Injection without pain- a child's right! Wow!

OBESITY AND HEALTH

Man or woman must weigh according to what their height permits and according to what the BMI (Body Mass Index) formula allows. BMI is equal to weight in kilograms divided by height in meters squared. If it is between 19.5 to 24.9 it is normal. If it is below the lower limit it is under-nutrition and if it is above 25, it is overweight until 29.9 and obesity after that.

Obesity is caused by not only over eating but also has some genetic predisposition in some cases. Obesity can cause many difficulties for the individual. Diabetes mellitus, hypertension, heart disease, respiratory disease like sleep apnoea, osteoarthritis of hip and knees are some of the problems that can be caused by obesity. Let's not forget the often associated psychological issues.

Weight loss is the only answer and it can be done by reducing calorie intake and increasing calorie output through exercise or combining both for good health and fitness.

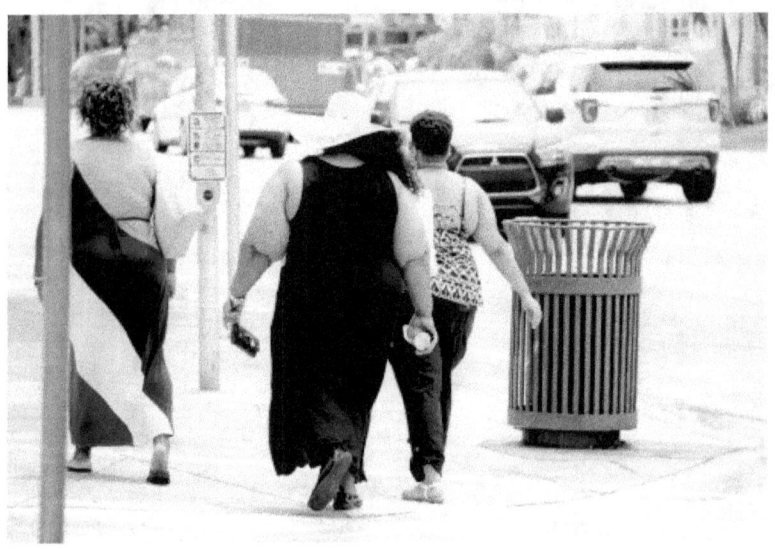

Adiposa Excessiva!

Folds of fat: Adiposa Excessiva!
Folds of fat, folds of fat,
Hanging from the chest, the waist and just below that,
Tell me dears, how on earth,

Did you quietly enter all places like that?
Folds of fat, you stores of fat,
Energy stored for a rainy day?
But that rain doesn't come the whole life long,
And we carry to grave the extra weight in pounds.
Laden with cholesterol and triglycerides,
Bloated become the fat cells-adipocytes!
From fatty streaks to atherosclerotic vessel plaques,
The organs get pale as the blood supply falls.
Measure it as body mass index or body weight,
Look for the shape of an apple or the pear shape!
Thickness of the Triceps fold will also show,
How much you need to stop to grow?
Lovely, beautiful, well rounded a person you make-
If at right places in right amounts you give a healthy state.
But hanging and bulging at wrong places,
You make one obese; give figureless, shapeless graces.
Children wonder, adults stare, give a naughty smile,
When the figure they see is elephantine.
The load is so much, the centre of gravity shifts,
Keeping in balance without a fall is hard, one drifts.
Giving large surface area, displacing large volume,
You help a person to float and swim,
But to walk or run on surface land,
Is like climbing Mount Everest without oxygen or wand.
Carrying the load of two or several in one,
The heart weeps silently, the knees cry aloud,
And the hips no longer can swing and dance,
To the rhyme and tune of the Song of Swan!
Folds and loads and tiers of fat, I know you,
And your secret routes and ways,
How easy to get the folds in place,
But how hard to melt you or displace.
Beware, behold, listen one and all,
There's only one way the thief can enter you all,

To rob you slowly but surely of,
Your figure, your shape, your health and all!
Two sweet lips surround its portal of entry,
The tongue that should guard is no more the sentry.
For the taste of sweets and fat it just won't detest,
When the thief's partner is the guard,
God save the owner and the landlord!
Lock your doors, friends, seal them well,
Train your guards of taste and smell,
For poison here is sweet, not bitter, and
Too much of a good thing is bad they tell.
Let's gird up our loins and make a resolve,
To watch our figures and keep us smart,
The balance of intake and output must show,
That more doesn't go in than we need to burn and glow.
Shapely figures of the fitness bums,
Envy of the young and of old dads and mums,
Let's cross the road to the fitness side,
And let them envy us in awe and surprise.
Wow, how beautiful!

-

OBESITY IS RELATED TO INTAKE AND OUTPUT IMBALANCE

-

Unless one has a rare metabolic disorder, it is all about calories ingested versus calories expended through work and exercise. If one has a positive calories balance, the excess accumulates in body's fat stores which almost have an unending capacity. There are some foods which are healthy for good physique, like a good mixture of fruits, vegetables, cereals, pulses, nuts and dry fruits. But there are certain foods which are good to taste but are dense in calories and poor in nutrition like minerals and vitamins. Examples of such foods are french fries and other fried oily stuff, chocolates, ice creams and milk shakes, butter and other sources of saturated fats. The fuel that we put in the body, we need to always keep a good watch on its quality and quantity.

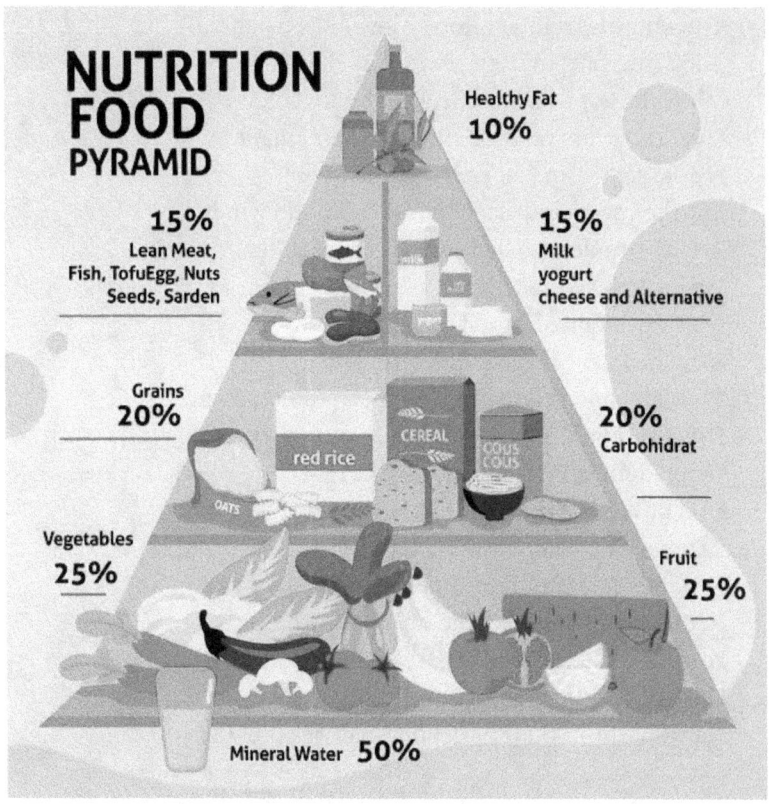

French fries, Burgers, Donuts, Milk shakes, ice creams etc high calorie density foods are missing from the Healthy Food Pyramid.

Fuel Watch!
Ronny was given charge of a machine,
That would take him places, run and swim.
He loved and adored it to a whim,
Always filled its tank to the brim!
Fuel in the machine was always in excess,
His travels consumed so much less.

Extra fuel got stored as lumps and bumps,
His machine became heavy, round and plump.
You know how much Ronny loved his machine,
Took care of it to the extent of a whim!
When he got it, it was sleek and buoyant,
Over the years he made it into a hefty giant.
It does take him places, as well as swim,
But the speed and alacrity is gone to the winds.
Ronny wonders as he looks at his machine,
He loved it so much yet it's failing him.
One day he met Uncle Quinn in a gym,
Who had kept his machine thin and slim!
"Too much love Son, needn't mean too much fuel,
Don't refill till it has consumed the first gruel."
"Fuel in must be equal to the fuel out,
Don't overfill now for a future drought!"
Ronny sadly had overfilled all his life,
Now he understood his uncle's precious advice.
He now runs his machine up and down,
Forces out stored fuel as sweat from his crown!
He watches the quantity and quality of fuel in,
He won't refill till the fuel out matches fuel in.

-

BRINGING BALANCE BETWEEN INTAKE AND OUTPUT

-

It is very important to keep one's weight within the limits allowed by one's height according to the charts and Body Mass Index within the normal range. Overweight and obesity are the causes of many ailments. Excess weight must be lost through reducing calories intake and increasing exercise through walking, jogging, running, gymming etc

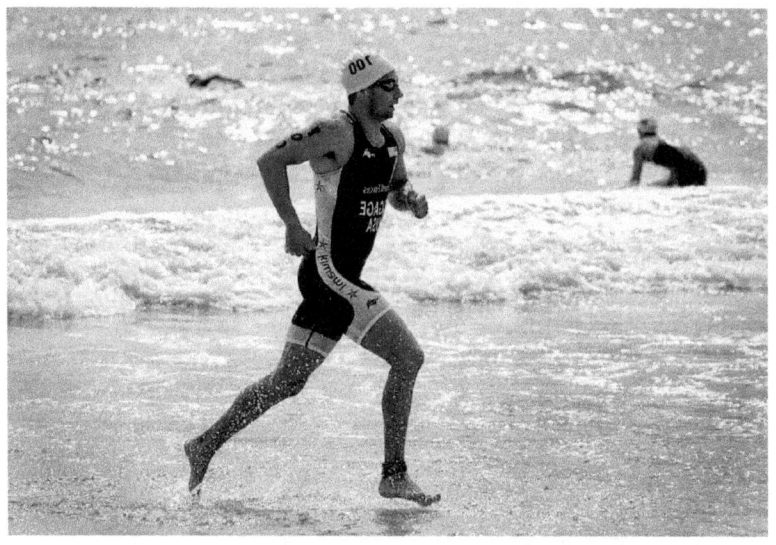

Fitness is a great feeling!

-

Lose, Lose!
If you lose your body's weight in ponds,
In case you are everywhere plump and round.
This loss will be your gain and triumph indeed,
You'll be healthier in word as well as in deed.
Losing flab in pounds is not for everyone a joke,
More so for those who love fast food and coke!
Wishing, wanting and hoping just won't work,
Determined drive alone gets you into slimmer shirt.
Puffing, panting, fuming and sweating,
By the roadside walking, running, as also jogging;
Straining and breaking your joints and bones,
You may try and lose those extra stones.
In gyms of hotels and flourishing health clubs,
Laboring on rowing machines, treadmill and stuff!
Dancing, jumping and huffing in aerobic classes,

You may lose some folds, some lumps, and some masses.
But lasting winners in this losing game,
Will be those who can also train and tame -
Taste buds on tongue, satiety center in the brain,
To eat less than what is needed for weight gain.
The sensitive balance of intake and drain,
We must achieve and also perpetually maintain.
So that having lost once, we don't regain,
Those shabby folds of fat and grain!
Dear myself! Come on dare yourself and lose,
This loss is going to be your gain profuse,
Fitness, smartness and no health care costs,
Are no mean gains to achieve and strive for!

-

WAIST HIP RATIO

-

Waist hip ratio is another measure of fitness or good health. If the waist girth increases more than the hips and the ratio goes from 0.8 to 0.9 to 1 or more, you are moving from good health to bad health. So watch your waist at all times! Increased waist girth is called central obesity. Central obesity is related to visceral or internal obesity which means fat surrounds the internal organs and chokes them as also the blood supply to the heart and other organs. Maintaing a slim waist is not only for the reason of beauty and fitness but it also means a lot for the health of internal organs and the heart.

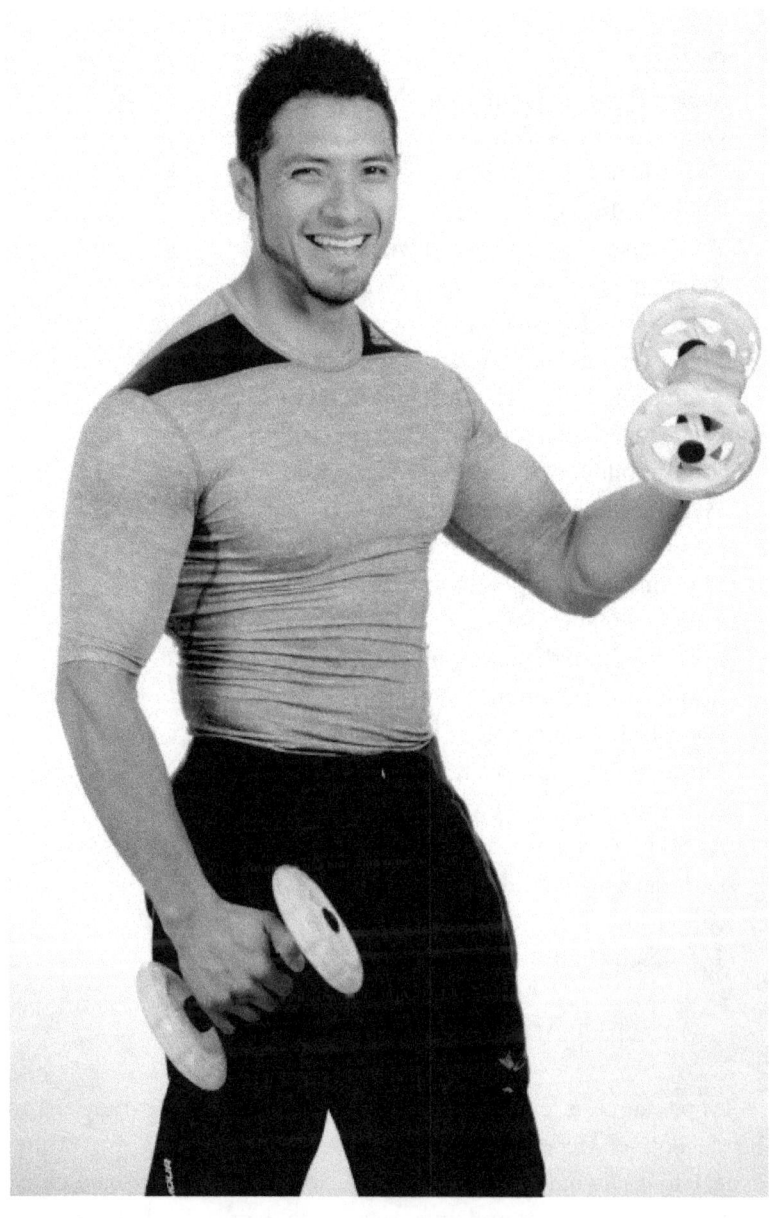

What a waist!

-

O Waist!

Waist, O Waist, O my dear, dear waist,
Once used to be slender, trim and sleek waist.
Could flaunt you freely in leisure or haste,
They used to ogle at you in such a great taste.
Food was then healthy and work was hard,
Keeping you slim was not such a big task.
Used to run to work and walk to shop,
That exertion kept you groomed in a shape tip-top.
Then came Pizza, fries and junk food of sorts,
I put them in my tummy as if it was a waste box.
Automobile took me everywhere without a trot,
Machines did all my chores and no sweat was lost.
Leisure time came in plenty, interesting TV to watch,
I became a couch potato munching chips as I watched.
These changing times and such changing lifestyles,
Brought about this plumpness that I dread to this while!
Results are so evident; my waist is now so vast,
I now only dream of that lean waist of my past.
I brought it upon myself; my great waist is lost,
Now they stare at my vast waist and feel aghast!
As they feel aghast they draw a lesson or two:
Let's eat only healthy, be energetic and active too!
Fatty foods are tasty poison our tongue gets used to,
Too much comfort is a bane, must start jogging too!

-

HAIR AND BEAUTY AND HEALTH

-

Appearance is everything. And yet they say appearances can be deceptive. Deceptive or otherwise, appearance is everything especially to a young man or woman. So many young people come to the clinic with complaints related to hair. The hairs are an appendage of the skin, so the skin specialist or dermatologist often attends to the hair problems. However some hair problems have basis in some hormone issues which must be looked in to. Almost all hair problems have associated psychological issues which too must be taken care of. Whereas some hair problems have answers, others have none.

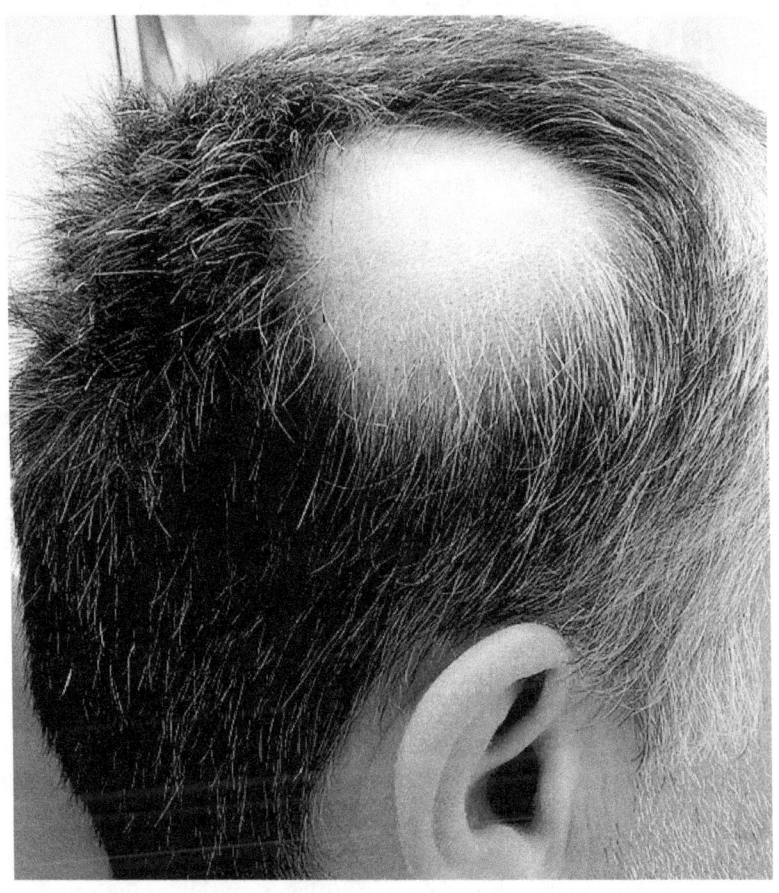

Hair loss is worrisome!

-
-
-

Mysterious Hair
You may have black or brunette, blonde or brown,
Straight and long, or short and curly on your crown!
Your hair mark you up, you may be a Dame or Sir,
Beauty, personality and identity are due to your hair, dear!
I was born with a plump and curly head of hair,
I'm not sure if I didn't take good care.
When my hair daily fell in big, big bunches,
I felt scared, full of cares; and I got bad hunches.
My hair was now here, now I see it nowhere,
Does anyone care? Please stop my falling hair!
It's going; it's gone for good, with the speed of a hare,
O my hair, my hair, my hair, my hair!
Mysterious Hair! It seems you don't care,
You deserted me and left my nice pate bare.
With you I was beautiful, even proud, O my dear,
Now I avoid public glare, for they laugh as they stare.
The doctors assured, if some hair fall, the others do grow,
Yet despite their hopes, my hair continued to go.
When most of it was gone, the doctors gave up pretences:
"Why we lose hair, Sir we fully don't know!"
A lady friend though had a different hair tangle,
She had more hair than what she loved to handle.
They grew at odd places she thought they made a scandal,
On her face, the trunk and on the legs above her ankles!
A doctor called it 'Hirsutism', did tests for various causes,
"No cause found; and not much to offer," he said with long
pauses.
She must shave them, cream them off, or undergo depilation,
She paid through her nose; her beautician was all jubilation!
A friend's hair became all grey, only in his twenties,
Something must be wrong, he saw doctors in plenty.
They accepted their ignorance without fanfare or fancy,
"About falling and graying of hair, our science is in infancy."
Mysterious hair - Forever mysterious hair!

DOCTOR, THERE IS TOO MUCH GAS IN ME

One of the very common complaints that all of us have is the problem of gas in the abdomen or stomach as they say. Quite often the doctor can not pin point the cause of the gas and quite often it is a very benign normal thing but some people are bothered too much by it. Doctors most often write some or the other medicine for indigestion, but some explaining is also required if it is being taken too seriously.

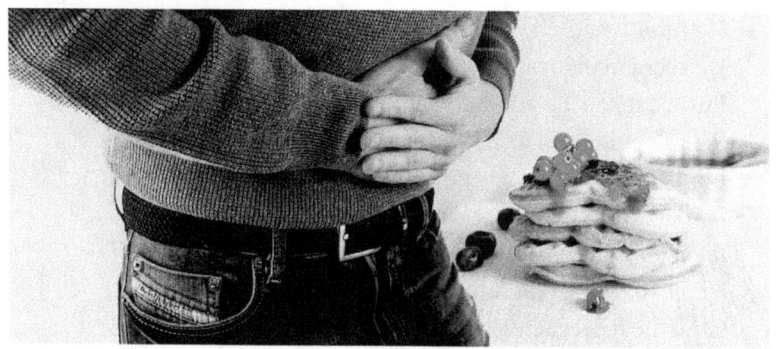

Food and dyspepsia or indigestion!

Gas factory!
Tom came to my clinic sullenly one day,
He was totally fed up with his gaseous ways!
He swore he ate - only solids and no gas,
And yet it seemed there was gas and only gas.
Gas, he felt filled his middle bloated section,
Gas also seeped from his top as well as bottom.
Burp and burp, turrr... and purr... was ever so often,
He couldn't rest or relax, it was incessant persistent.
The mid-segment gurgles and the musical borborygmi,

Were heard by his friends who smiled and looked funny!
The burps and the turrps were so noisy and boisterous,
They stopped strangers who gave looks not innocuous.
He described his predicament with near tears in his eyes,
To what length he went to avoid public's ears and eyes.
He always looked for corners to let the gas pass,
He would often turn the tap to drown the noise of the gas.
He tilted right or left to make way for the gas,
He first looked around to let the passer-by pass.
This explosive gas problem had made his life a shambles,
He thought people laughed wherever he assembled.
This gas had made him nuts, his life was miserable,
He felt he had no control and that made him depressed.
He recognized some foods as gas-makers notorious,
But whatever he ate ended up in this gas so mysterious!
What could I tell Tom I was in a dilemma and quandary?
I looked into his eyes and told him this truth extra-ordinary:
"O dear, don't you feel lonely; nor do you feel depressed,
It's every guy's problem, so you now cheer up instead!"
He heard with rapt attention how the gas was formed,
How the 'Gas Factory' worked in our body's mid-land.
How dangerous it would be if the gas stopped to come!
So finally he smiled and said to the gas, 'Welcome!'

-

HEART HEALTH- ANGINA PECTORIS

-

One very common ailment of the heart is the narrowing of the heart's blood vessels or coronary arteries that get narrowed due to wall thickening caused by atherosclerosis and resulting in reduced blood supply to heart muscle producing chest pain called angina pectoris. The process of atherosclerosis is progressive and age related and is promoted by high Blood Pressure, Diabetes Mellitus, high blood Cholesterol, Smoking, Sedentary lifestyle and Stress with a background of family history. It can be delayed by taking care of these modifiable risk factors.

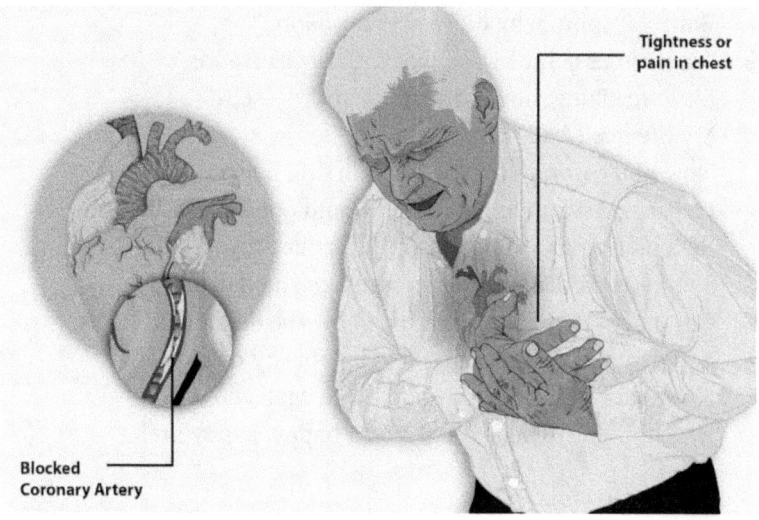

Tightness or pain in chest

Blocked Coronary Artery

Chest pain or angina is due to blockage of heart's blood supply!

-

Angina- Stable to Unstable
How is your angina, Mr. John?
"It was quite stable, Sir, for so very long,
Chest pain would come if I walked 200 yards,
I would hold my chest and rest, and it would pass.
I would use a tablet under the tongue to climb or go far,
I knew my coronaries well, until a fortnight, Sir.
Now day and night, walking little, or even at rest,
They bring out a sweat, don't let me rest.
May God help me, now the tablet doesn't help,
My unstable coronaries now constantly protest.
"Dear John, you know there is an atherosclerotic plaque,
It gets fissured slightly and is called the ruptured plaque..
Platelets and fibrin would have made a clot on its top,
Already narrow vessels were thus, further blocked.
Blood supply to the heart's muscle got further jeopardized,

Heart muscle suffered ischemia and with chest pain you cried."
But Dear John, why did you take so long?
"Foolishness, Sir, I was busy with life's errands,
Little realizing, how on such narrow vessels,
My life itself had hanged!"
Now don't worry John, you are in safe hands,
Heparin, Aspirin and Nitrates would open blocked bands.
Beta blockers and Dilzem would reduce myocardial demands,
Soon you would once again stabilize and dance!
Coronary Angiography would show the degree of blocks,
You may then opt to have an Angioplasty or Bypass.
No shouting coronaries then, no struggle, no strife,
And hopefully then, you'll lead a happy, happy life!

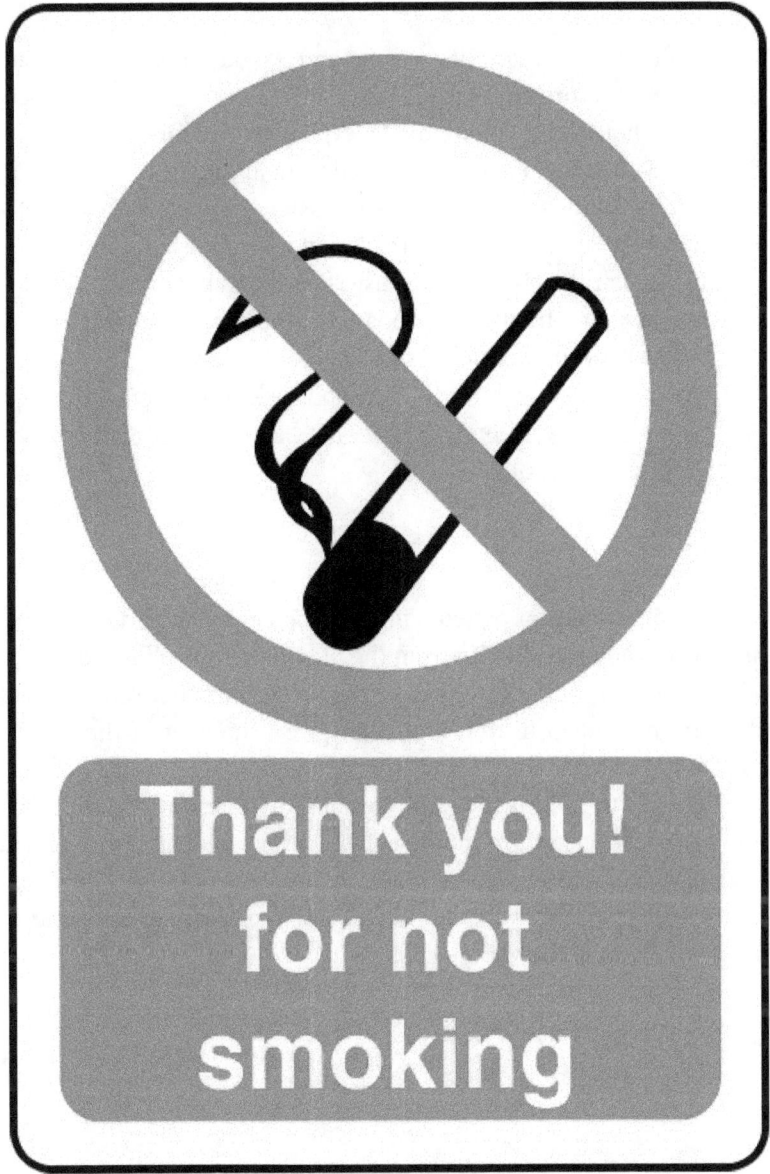

Smoking- active and even passive, is a serious risk factor for angina. Stopping smoking quickly brings down the chances of another attack.

Within 20 minutes, heart rate and blood pressure start to decrease and return back to normal

After 8 hours carbon monoxide levels start to drop

After 24 hours, ability to smell and taste improves

After 72 hours breathing becomes easier

After 2 weeks to 3 months circulation improves

After 1 year the risk of heart disease is cut in half

After 15 years the risk of coronary heart disease is similar to that of individuals who have never smoked.

https://www.williamoslerhs.ca/about-osler/news-media/live-well-with-osler/safety-prevention/what-happens-to-your-body-when-you-quit-smoking

-

ALCOHOL AND MAN'S HEALTH

-

A good number of patients in a doctor's clinic in certain places are those who are suffering from the ill effects of alcohol addiction. These people got into alcohol for fun or tension relief remedy, but they are now deep in to it and can't give it up even if they want to. That is addiction. They and their families suffer but addictions are not easy to quit. It requires specialised clinics for de-addiction and these services are not available everywhere. There is an organization called, 'Alcoholic Anonymous' which also helps but is not available everywhere. Alcohol that most people consume is chemically Ethanol or Ethyl alcohol.

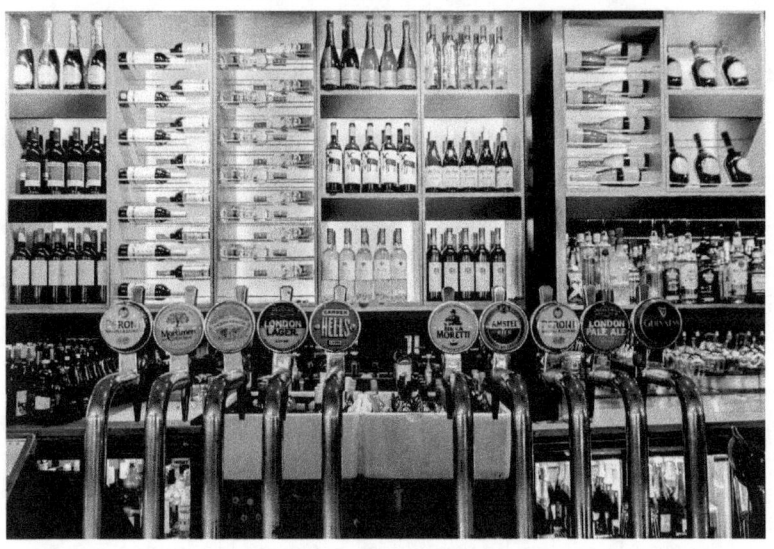

The very respectable pub!

-

<u>O Ethanol!</u>
Ethanol, Ethanol; some people love you, Ethanol,
You're life and soul of the pub, Ms. Ethanol!
To lose inhibitions and communicate well,
They sit and chat with friends, on Ethanol.
The 'high', the 'kick' and the 'tipsy' feeling,
They love you for all that, O Ethanol.
You drown their sorrows, for the moment fleeting,
You make them forget themselves, Ethanol.
Now, you have the Doctor's stamp of approval,
"It protects from heart attacks," Saint Ethanol!
Fourteen units a week for ladies, twenty one for gentlemen-
Is the dose advised by even the Royal College of Physicians!
But neurons in the brain, they ask for more,
To limit the amount is no small chore,
The good feeling it gives, many want of it more,

In the flood of more they drown, can't swim ashore.
In no time then 'habituation' sets in,
'Dependence' on Ethanol follows soon,
'Addiction then holds them in its firm grasp,
Devoid of will power one is helpless in its clasp.
Bereft of will power what is man?
His health to him is of no consequence.
Ethanol mercilessly destroys his organs.
Liver, heart and brain, consider lost and gone.
But Ethanol destroys not only the man,
His loving family's fate is also sealed in 'the can'.
Ethanol is a saint with a fiendish hidden side,
Its luring glances are deceptive; don't you commit suicide!
Stay away; Stay away friend, from this unnatural balm,
Or else be the next victim on Ethanol's palm.
Beware! Don't try; be wary of its power and influence,
Be in self-control, live in original glory and natural countenance!
-

DRUG ADDICTION IS KILLING: STAY AWAY
-

There are all kinds of addicting substances like opium, heroin, cocaine, marijuana etc available in the social circles. Young people are falling a prey to this savage attraction and they are losing their youth and chances of doing anything worthwhile in their lives. It is so very painful for a doctor to see. The latest fad in US is the e-cigarette among school students and youngsters. It is supposed to contain nicotine and was meant as Nicotine replacement therapy for smokers but it became available to youngsters and they have gotten addicted to it. And because of contaminants in it, dozens of young people have died after developing pneumonia after inhaling the e cigarette smoke which is also called vaping.

But again, a doctor is too small a fry to stop the social aspects of the problem like smuggling and sales of these substances. He can only hope to advise and help through de-addiction clinics! In a state of addiction advice does not work. A long process of de-addiction has to be undergone by a willing person. Advice works possibly for those who are not yet into it or only just trying out.

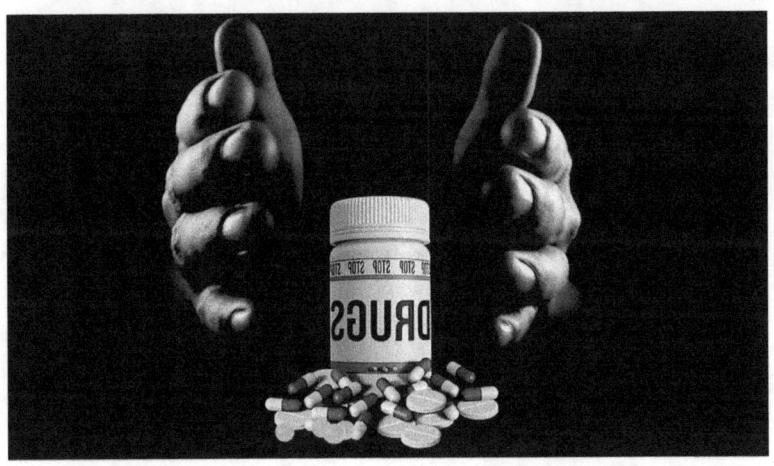

No, no, no: Say no to drugs!

No, No, No; Say No to Drugs!
It started as fun, with the Devil's friendly gesture,
Who offered a free 'kick', a "high", a heavenly pleasure,
Resisted for a time, but succumbed to 'peer pressure',
Tasted temptation a few times and got hooked in full measure.
Free offer withdrawn, had to pay for every kick,
Beg or steal, someone's soles he would lick,
Need was great, would do anything, for the needle prick,
Devilish friends deserted, created one more addict.
Work, study and relations, dwindled and suffered,
Lived like a beggar, life in penury, lay shattered!
No happiness, no cheer, only misery, fear and pain,
Life revolved around Morphine, Heroin and Cocaine.
One bad habit, brings other worse vices,
Bad Company made him unsocial; only criminal choices,
He cared for nothing but his transitory pleasure,

He was sought by law, in search of a treasure.
Whom to blame for the mess he is in,
Himself, his parents, his company, or genes?
The addict has brought his life to a ruin,
Strangers too cry, to see the end of a dream!
Beware, beware, beware O young one!
Choose your company with care and far vision,
Take parents', teachers', well-wishers' guidance,
Sort out right and wrong, with their love & assistance.
Stay on right track; seek real fun and progress,
Stick firmly to right, don't waver or transgress,
Say a firm 'no' to drugs and boosters today,
Live on inner happiness for the rest of your days.

ROAD TRAFFIC ACCIDENTS AND THE DOCTOR

When posted in Accident and Emergency department of the hospital, a doctor comes across a lot of pain. One of the very unfortunate causes of this pain are the road traffic accidents which kill and maim many a young persons. Road traffic accidents or RTAs as they are called happen due to many causes, some of which are speeding, drunken driving, sleep deficit - sleeping while driving, angry or post emotional injury driving, texting while driving, phoning while driving- these are some of the driver related issues which cause accidents. There can be road quality related issues and inadequacy of light related issues, animals crossing the road suddenly, and poor visibility due to rain, fog or storm- all these can be the cause of road accidents. A doctor in the emergency room can only take good care of the injured patient, but this is the most preventable cause of morbidity and mortality and society needs to take care of it, each one of us have to be safe drivers and follow the rules of the road and land.

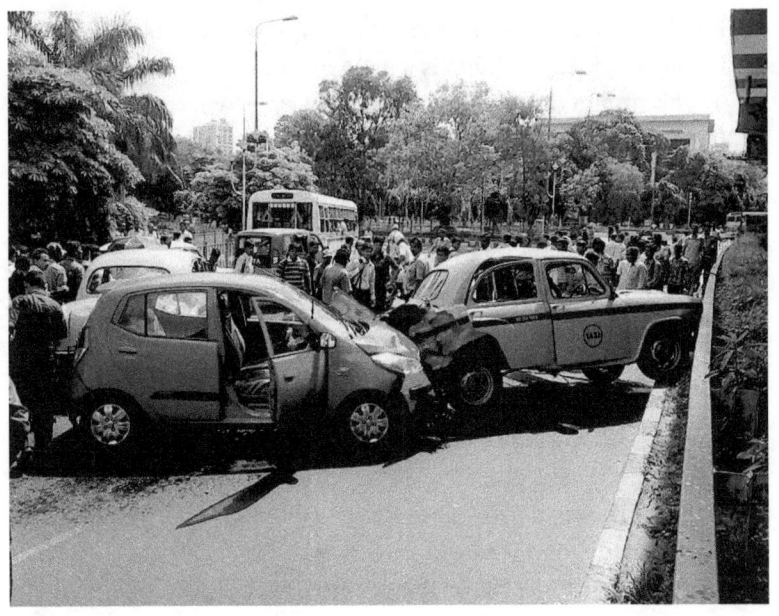

Drive carefully with 100% attention for safety!

-

<u>Dangerous Moves</u>
If you enter somehow a 'No entry' zone,
To the fellow from the other side, you're not known.
Your move is full of consequences known and unknown,
Avoid this dangerous move; be you novice or well known.
You're young at heart; you've a love of thrill,
You love to talk with the winds, cross speeds with a shrill.
Your machine may give way without notice or drill,
Speeding is a dangerous move; it may disable or kill.
You're a funny guy, love to chat on the wheel,
Either on your phone or with those in the automobile!
You may lose your focus; shift your eyes from the road,
Dangerous to lose control, dear keep a good hold.
You great guy, you think your Dad's are the roads,

Why other users and why pedestrians cross the road?
But do know better, roads are for everyone's sensible use,
Being oblivious of others is a dangerous move.
'Drinking and driving don't mix' they everywhere say;
Inebriated you feel great but you zigzag and sway.
You may drive on but you misjudge at every step,
Make not this dangerous move, you better give up.
"I'll wear no helmet; I love no seat belt,
Don't curb my freedom, I'm a free bird."
To stay free dear, you must be safe at first,
No dangerous moves; follow safety rules with trust.
Didn't sleep well or took drugs to fall asleep?
Driving with droopy eyes dear how will you peep?
If not fully awake don't leave your homestead,
It's a dangerous move you better be rested instead.
'A million die on the world's roads every year,'1
So 2004 was the WHO's "Road Safety Year." 2, 3
Each one of us must shun all the dangerous moves,
For 'the largest and most preventable epidemic' to be removed!
4.

-

References:

1One million people die on world's roads every year.Owen Dyer. British Medical Journal (BMJ) 2004, April 10,328: 851.

2.**Road Traffic injury prevention**. Barry Pless. Editorial. BMJ 2004, April 10, 328: 846

3.**War on the roads: two years on**. Ian Roberts, Kamran Abbasi. Editorial. BMJ 2004, April 10, 328: 845.

4. **Road safety advocacy**. Jeanne Breen. Education and Debate. BMJ 2004, April 10, 328: 888-890

-

MAN AGAINST MAN

-

Man has no patience, man is very angry, man is very quick to blame, man is almost eager to fight in order to hopefully save himself through fighting or at least prove a point to the other person. All these parameters are applicable when an accident happens on the road between two parties and the immediate result is a road rage between them and sometimes it can be more serious than the original accident and rarely the rage itself ends in fatality. Quite a sad state of affairs!

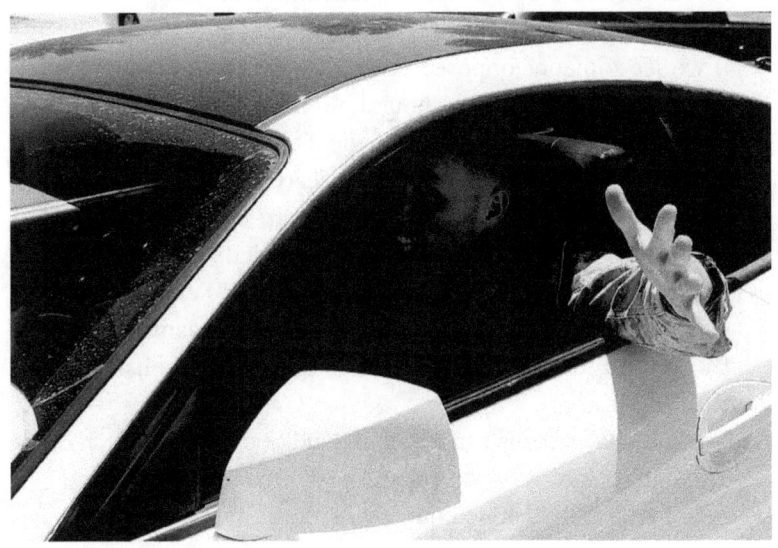

Control your anger on the road!

Road Rage

A car just touched and scratched another car yesterday,
The drivers came out and fought till one was dead that day.
This is not the first time such a deadly thing has happened,
This fit of rage called 'road-rage', on roads it often happens.
We keep our anger handy, ready to use and roll,
So, quickly it bursts out and goes out of our control.
In the clash of egos, each declares: 'You wrong, me right.'
We often find it easy to yell at another and fight.
We carry so much intolerance of others built within,

We start abusing and blaming others for faults so thin.
When our hearts are full of irritation, hate and defiance,
At the drop of a hat we start screaming in annoyance.
In this competitive world and it's fast paced life,
Selfishness reigns and we are full of stress and strife.
Goals are so important; means have lost their meaning,
So our actions are selfish, intolerant and demeaning.
We harbor strong views and opinions; likes and dislikes,
If we see someone opposed, we revolt, we just don't like.
If opposition is weak, we shout, fight and strike,
If opposition is strong, we often yield and keep quiet.
We claim we are full of love in our hearts,
But our love is superficial and selective to start.
Our love is limited to few; most are excluded from our hearts,
So we boil easily when hit by even a stranger's cart.
On the road, when accident has happened and damage is done,
By blaming the other, we try to lessen our responsibility and burden.
We take law into our hands; accuse, judge and punish each other,
The fight goes out of control and both are bound to suffer.
In some societies police quickly arrives; there's no use for any rage,
Where law is not so prompt, you live with a lot of road rage.
If one party remains quiet and generous, doesn't get into a rage,
Both may then be lucky to survive the deadly worm of road rage.

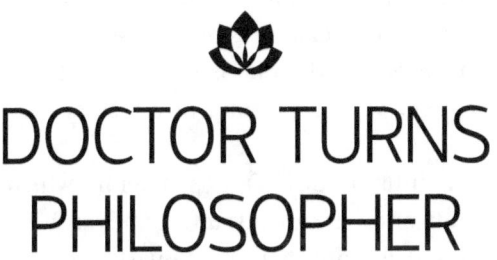

CHAPTER FIVE

DOCTOR TURNS PHILOSOPHER

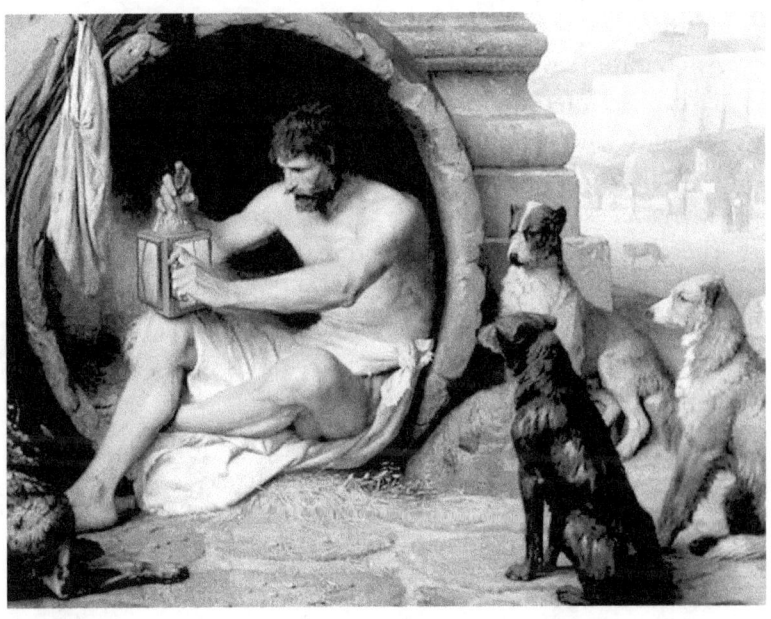

Diogenes - The Greek Philosopher, sitting in his tub. Painting by Jean-Leon Jerome. 1860 CE.When Alexander went to meet Diogenes and exhorted him to ask for anything from him, he replied, " You are blocking my sunlight, please just get to one side."

THE SAD STORY OF MAN

Man, although top in the animal kingdom, yet is not the master of it which he sometimes claims to be after small successes in small ventures. Every now and then he is made to feel small in front of Nature and its very wide repertoire of disasters troubling man in million ways.

The Corona Virus or COVID 19 pandemic which is currently going on in the world has already infected over 20 million people worldwide and killed more than three quarters of a million people in just 6 months. Man is very vulnerable. He is humbled every now and then by Mother Nature.

Vulnerable man!

Earthquakes, tornadoes, typhoons and blizzards,
Are Nature's severe convulsions, and man's deadly hazards!
Volcanoes, infernos, hurricanes and floods,
Man looks meager in front of Nature's mighty spread.
An ant-bite, a bee-sting, a scorpion or a snake's bite,
A jelly-fish sting, a spider-bite, can all take a man's life.
These small but visible dangers threaten the existence of man,
Invisible microbes make a mockery of the pride of man.
Yet man is so arrogant, whenever he begins to talk,
Feels all powerful as if Master of all Nature's stock.
It's true his spirit can't be killed or oppressed,
His body is too delicate and weak in fact.
Man is so susceptible, incapable of his defense,
Now he is bragging, next moment he's across life's fence.
Is he the spirit or the body, who is the real man?
Invincible spirit with vulnerable body, this combo is man!

NATURE IS SO POWERFUL YET SO EQUAL

Natural calamities can uproot a man in seconds and yet it does not choose between all the differences men have created on this earth to separate man from man. Besides created differences of geography, nationality, skin color, caste and creed, the greatest of them is religion, where each religion claims to be the best and true knower of God. But does God favor that religion in any way?

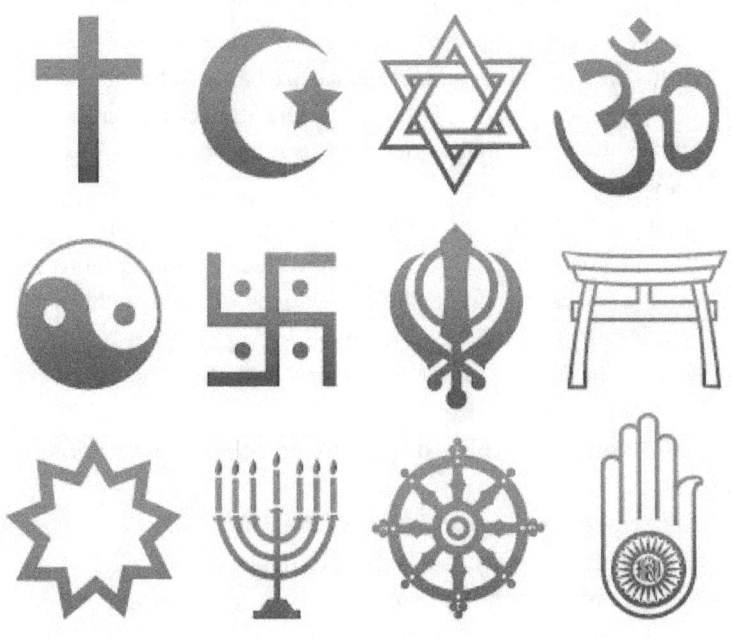

Different religions: Just One Humanity!

-

God's Favorite!
I don't know why each religion's followers are taught,
That theirs' is the best and direct from God.
That all the rest are at best a useless lot:
"They ought to be taught and into 'our' fold brought."
They talk of God as Omnipotent, Omnipresent and Omniscient;
But limit and confine Him with their every thought and act.
"We are His favourites and know God as nobody else,
To him the hell who doesn't believe like us!"

I don't know why such preachers fail to learn,
From Nature, which is not human but God's own!
Their fixed ideas don't loosen their grasp,
Their ingrained views blind their whole lot.
Tsunami* of 26 December 2004 was an eye opener indeed-
God would kill without favouring any faith or creed.
Thousands of Indonesian Muslims, Sri-Lankan Buddhists,
Christians in Thailand, Hindus in India all perished en-masse!
All religions are equally good and each has its bad,
They should see humanity as one, as does God!
Creating differences among humans on religious basis is bad,
Those who do so, I wonder, if they've really understood God.
You may stick to your religion, in which you're brought up,
That is your life-line; you mustn't give it up.
But for God's sake, don't consider other religions' followers as fools,
Even though they pray differently and their ways are not that cool.
If preachers teach brotherhood of their own fellows - it is great,
It'll be greater if they taught Brotherhood of Man without hate.
Natural brotherhood of man cuts across religions and states,
Man's destiny is sealed in Unity and together we meet Tsunami's fate!

-

Tsunami*: A Japanese word for a very forceful sea-wave which starts from the site of an under-sea earthquake and spreads peripherally in all directions at speeds of over 300-400 miles an hour and on reaching the shores its speed lessens but the height increases up to 10 meters. It swallows and extinguishes all life on shore where thousands perish in no time as in the latest Tsunami of 26th December 2004 when the human toll crossed two hundred fifty thousand with maximum damage done in Indonesia, Sri Lanka, India, Thailand and Africa when the epicenter lay around the Indonesian island of Sumatra.

-

NATURAL DISASTERS DEVASTATE MAN
-

Droughts, floods, earthquakes, volcano eruptions, hurricanes, cyclones, typhoons, lightning, tsunamis they come suddenly and destroy a man in no time. All of man's dreams of a good life and great future come to a naught in no time. Man is indeed vulnerable. Running, running, running faster then is of no avail when a wave of tsunami is following you, as happened in the Japanese Tsunami of 2011.

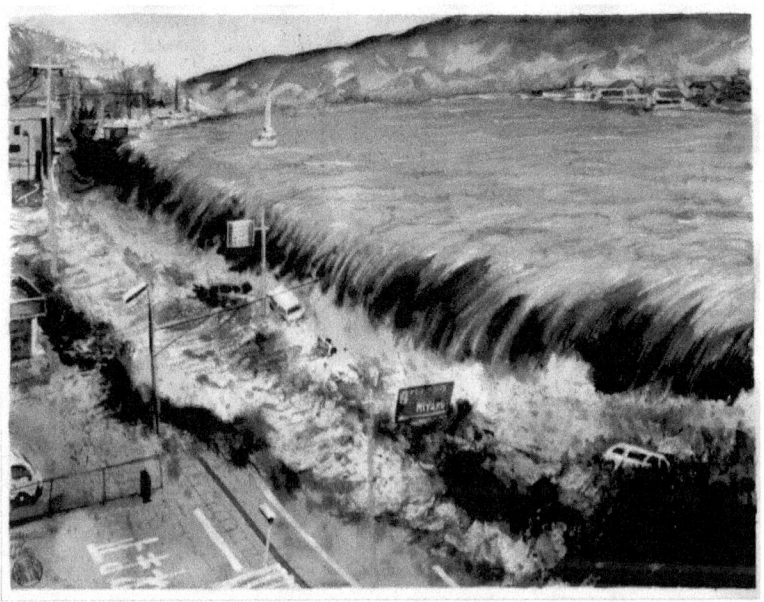

The fierce power of the sea in Tsunami!

-

<u>Gone in a moment- Japanese Tsunami 2011</u>
You build your future bit by bit by bit,
You build your house brick by brick by brick.
You build your life day in and day out,
You build on what you think is solid ground.

You build and you think it'll stay for good,
You hope to stay in it for as long as you could.
You build and create for your family in style,
You do your best so you may live in style.
You may build for good but don't be fooled,
Seeing the Japanese Tsunami I'm no more fooled.
On March 11, 2011, after a 9.0 earthquake in the ocean,
A strong Tsunami wave came running to land from ocean.
10 meter high, half a kilometer wide running at 800Km/Hr speed,
Nothing could stand and nothing stayed in front of that wave indeed.
Thousands of houses, cars, trucks, boats were uprooted and tossed as toys,
The powerful wave kept going for 10 Km inland and destroyed these toys.
There was a warning to run but the twenty minutes time was short to run,
Only a few could escape and many were caught in the speeding ocean.
The exact toll of human lives lost in not exactly known till a week,
Over 10,000 casualties are predicted; situation is grim, heart weak.
Those who survived, saw destruction all around, their everything was lost,
Affluent until yesterday, they were rendered homeless; lived at community's cost.
One survivor who lost all, said she doesn't know if it was good or bad to survive,
The devastation and destruction was so much watching it even on TV some cried.
You're making big plans for future, you may, but do beware in this world,

And do prepare yourself for anything happening at any time in this world.

Nature is very powerful, very dramatic and can often give you surprises,

Be mentally ready for the worst, so you don't get astounded by its surprises.

-

WITNESSING DEATH

As a doctor, encounter with death and dying patients gives goose bumps often. Death of a patient can sometimes be a very emotionally draining experience for the doctor. Especially if the doctor had been treating the patient and had known the family of the patient, it can be a traumatic experience for him. Under such circumstances giving solace to the family is another function that the doctor must undertake. Also sometimes it can be very difficult explaining to the family the circumstances of the patient's death. It can be very challenging.

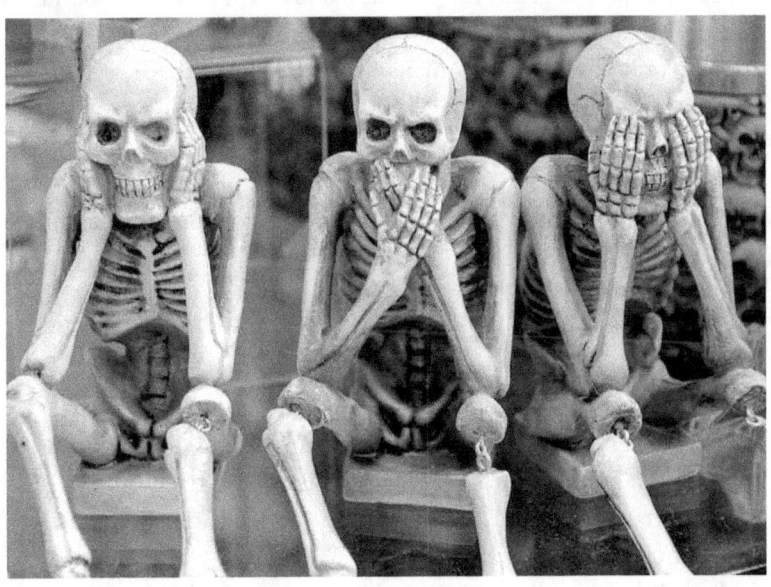

See no evil, hear no evil and speak not evil, so say the bones!!

-

<u>Till Death do us apart!</u>

Fifty eight point eight million die every year on planet earth*,

The World Health Organization** testifies the grim dance of death.

Death appears to be inevitable and compulsory in the life of man,

I had almost forgotten it; come to think of it, O man! O man!

Why doesn't it seem near? Why doesn't it feel real? That is a wonder,

Why are we oblivious of it? So impervious to the idea of it; it's a wonder.

I feel as if I am here forever; I hope by a flick of chance I may see of it never,

I love it how it is; I wish I could be the one who stayed here forever, forever.

The scenery is great, the weather is lovely; I love the mountains and the valleys,

The buildings and the mansions are grand; there are joyous crowds in the alleys.

Come home and the wife is loyal, kids are obedient and caring, the dog is loving;

Everything is in plenty, who would like to leave this world, O my! It is bewitching!

God is great; bank balance is full, business is flourishing; there are friends galore,

People love me, they call me great; heavens are kind, I am successful to the core.

The thought of leaving this never comes to me; such talk or even thought is a bore,

I never can think all this may one day end; mine, I feel is an ongoing chore.

I don't believe them when looking at my grey hair they call me old,

I know I'm young; I'm young at heart; those who think they are old are old.

I'm stuck; I'm stuck; I'm firmly stuck to this world with a heart of gold,

Its attraction has entered my heart and soul; I'm you know not yet too old.

Well, well, well; the WHO statistics are too sharp, biting and disheartening,

It seems I'll have to think of the unthinkable; howsoever bore and frightening.

I can either dumbly wait for my turn and grow dull, duller and depressed;

Or be prepared to go and yet live each day in thankfulness and feel blessed.

-

*Anthony S Fauci, David M Moreans. The Perpetual Challenge of Infectious Diseases; New England Journal of Medicine: 2012, Feb2; 366, 454-61

** World health statistics 2011. Geneva: World Health Organization, 2011.

-

THE BEGINNINGS OF NEW LIFE

-

How does life originate? Life has been there since eternity. How does a new form originate? That is the question that a doctor is taught in a subject called Embryology and related to this is the science of Genetics or the study of genes. It is genes which decide what will be the color of your iris and skin, your height and stature and many or all other features and contours that you call yours. There is a science of origin of the form as is there of origin of species according to Darwin's laws of evolution. We learn and see that all of us have similar origins.

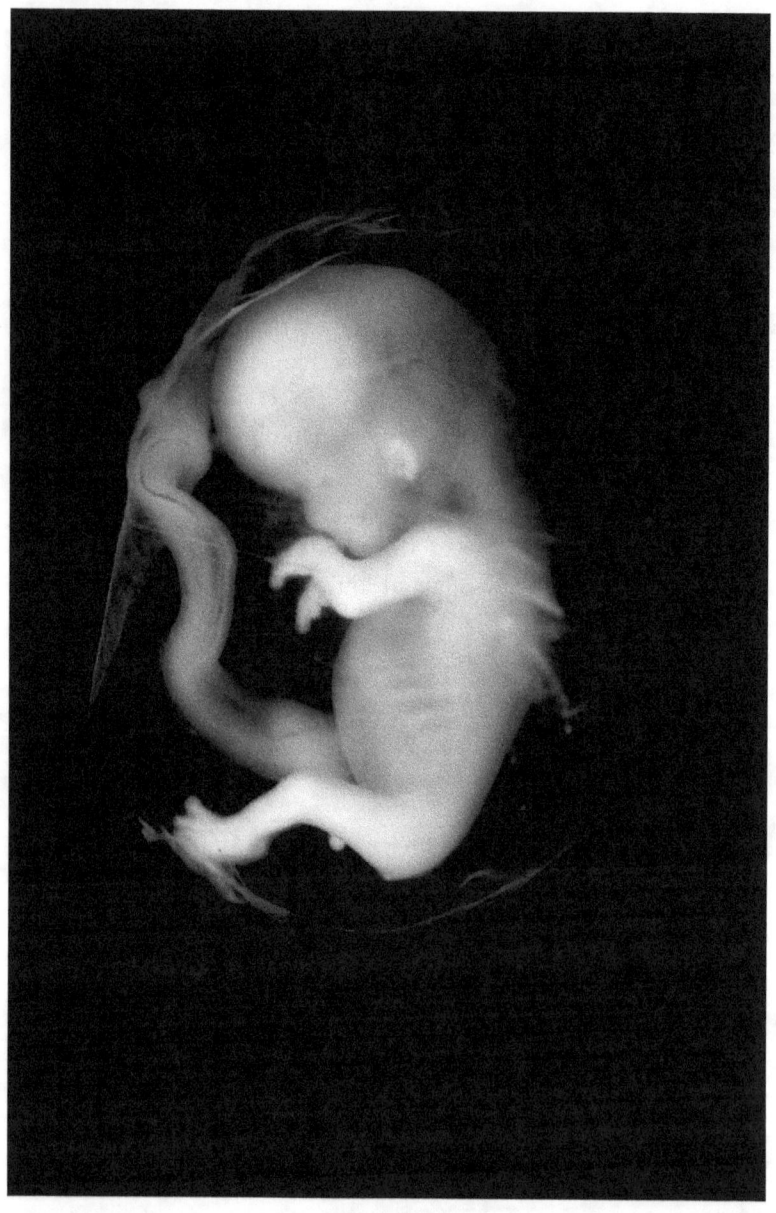

The beginning of a new life!

-

Our common origins!

How far back you can go in tracing your lovely story?

When you were born and cried, is that where begins your story?

With loud cries you moved about your limbs, is that the real start?

No, no, no; that's much later; that's too gross a start!

You didn't have any limbs; neither did you have any parts,

You won't recognize yourself at all; well that is how you start.

On a Science T.V channel the other day, technology opened my eyes,

How a boy or a girl comes into being, it was quite a surprise.

Scene one; millions and millions of mouse like guys with a winding tail,

They were jumping around as if in a competitive race on a forest trail.

It seemed each so very well knew its direction and destination,

They called them 'sperms', well that was their scientific designation.

Scene two; The ovary releases a round sort of 'spry'they called an 'ovum',

This one headed quietly towards the fallopian tube to meet someone its own.

One of the sperms was very smart and fast, was the first to arrive in the tube,

There it met and joined the ovum; the two became one in that narrow tube.

The ovum quickly put a block on seeing and meeting any other guests,

Whatever happened to other millions of sperms; they died in the race I guess.

Scene three: The story now is focused on the conjoined ovum and sperm,

They called it a 'zygote'; within it were left the chromosomes of the sperm.

Half the chromosomes came from ovum and half from the sperm,

The zygote had double the number plus an X or a Y from the sperm.

If the sperm was X and joined the X of the ovum, you will have a XX girl,

If the sperm was Y and joined the ovum's X, you'll be a XY boy not a girl.

Now with the full diploid chromosome number, the zygote became very active,

This one cell divides to become two, then four, eight, sixteen at a speed superlative.

This bunch of cells starts moving from the tube to the cavity called the 'uterus',

This 'Oocyst' gets implanted to grow in the spacious cavity of the uterus.

Scene four: The next nine months will be spent here in this cozy uterine cavity,

They showed how the spine got formed; eyes appeared far apart on the face in reality.

The brain then formed, the limbs sprout up; fingers and toes then came up,

The head was too big, bigger than any other part and then the genitals showed up.

They showed very beautifully how now the heart starts beating and the limbs go kicking,

You started moving the fingers as if grasping and at times in your nose you were picking.

This growing 'you', 'the fetus', enveloped by a sac was connected to the cord umbilicus,

All nutrition for the rapidly growing 'you' came from the mother through this umbilicus.

Scene five: Nine months over and the uterus starts contracting to get you out into the world,

This is how the story was told, of how long you took to get ready for the outside world.

So you started as a single cell called a 'zygote'; made half from ovum and half from sperm,

Remember, at your origin you were a mere cell, not as you claim, a man or a woman.

Are you then just a bundle of cells indeed? And what happens when someone dies?

The bundle of cells remains but what has gone missing? Missing is the one who said, 'I', 'I';

The energy, the life, you remember that was in the hyperactive sperm and the ovum,

That energy or electricity in each is the 'I'; not the cells or the form of every man or woman.

A million different types of electric bulbs, give differing lights hanging from an electric wire,

When one bulb fuses, it is useless and dead; but electricity keeps running in the ever live wire.

Dead bulbs get removed and new ones are put; the current of life goes on and on,

Your body may go but 'you' the energy will go on; you may spring up in a brand new form!

-

BREATH IS LIFE

-

We all depend on a breath of air for our survival from birth when we take our first breath and until we take our last breath. Breath of air gives us the very vital oxygen required for the function of the brain and other vital organs. A human being can survive without taking a breath ordinarily for no more than 2-3 minutes, although some people through breath holding training can do it a little longer.

This process of breathing must start soon after a baby's birth or else.......

-

<u>The other umbilicus</u>
When a baby comes out of the mother's womb,
The umbilical cord is cut and tied,
The baby utters a vehement cry,
All is well, everyone is happy and smiles.
But, if the baby is born and wouldn't cry,
The hue turns blue, Apgar* score is three or two,
The doctor fervently taps its back and sucks the throat dry,
To make it cry.
Troubled by the beating and the irritation,
The baby emits an angry, incessant cry,
The colour turns to pink, the baby is active and spry,
Apgar is now ten, the doctor is relieved and smiles.
With the first cry, goes in the first breath of air,
Which blows in life - the most vital oxygen of air.
For, when one umbilical cord is cut,
The other must soon connect,
Just to keep the life in motion.
If somehow, the other cord, the breath, failed to connect,
Within minutes, the Apgar would fall from three to naught,
The colour would turn from blue to black.
The fuse would blow, life would cease to glow.
The other umbilical cord, made of linear breaths of air,
Hangs us through our mouths and noses,
To the womb of Mother Nature;
This vital connection must go on and on,
As long on, as life itself goes on.
We all hang on to our One Mother Nature,
With the same umbilical cord, the breath,
Believe it or not, the truth remains for all to see,
We are the children of the same Mother; and hence Brothers!

-

* Apgar score: a measure of the physical condition of a newborn infant. It is obtained by adding points (2, 1, or 0) for heart rate, respiratory effort, muscle tone, response to stimulation, and skin coloration; a score of ten represents the best possible condition.

THE CYCLE OF LIFE

We are born; we grow, we degenerate and we die. The cycle has been going on since times immemorial and there is no respite from it for anyone, big or small, rich or poor, king or commoner. On seeing this cycle, anyone can become philosophical but a doctor knowing the cycle from close quarters becomes not only philosophical but also very realistic. He tries to develop a balanced attitude and a sense of equanimity and calmness towards the phenomena of life.

From One Cavity to Another

We begin our journey in the mother's womb,
A cavity that keeps us cosy for nine months long!
The zygote divides into two, then four, in a regular fashion,
When the 'Soul' enters, is still a matter of speculation!
We then grow and grow till we nearly fill the cavity,
When it can't hold us, we exit it with force and gravity.
From a cosy, small cavity, into such a wide open space,
It's irritating at first, but love makes it a liveable place!
This place, this world, this wide planet earth,
Is but a small object in the wider Universe!
In this world too, our sizes and numbers grow,
We build cosy houses as cavities to live and glow.
We grow, travel, talk, learn and get wise-
"And so, from hour to hour, we ripe and ripe,
And then, from hour to hour, we rot and rot,
And thereby hangs a tale", so the Bard of Avon* taught.
Our journey begun does come to an end,
From a cavity begun, into a cavity it ends.

When the live world can't hold us any more,
We enter another cavity, the grave, for eternal rest-
From where we'll be forced out nowhere, no more!
* Bard of Avon = William Shakespeare: in "As you Like It".

-

WHAT IS MAN?

It's a difficult question: What is man? Some suggest asking the question from oneself: Who am I? Again, it is not an easy question to find the answer to. But we should make a try! Ordinary observation of life and people shows that all of us can be of several different combinations of good, bad and ugly depending upon which part of our multi faceted nature gets activated at a particular time. It is however difficult to judge and the wise also reccommend: 'Judge Not!'

-

'Intel inside!
On every personal computer (PC) you see today,
'Intel Inside' is embossed on its bay.
'Intel' make the chip that makes the PC work,
Without the chip the PC is mere trash, won't work!
Human body is a super computer in every way,
It works day in and out in a near perfect way.
What is in it? I looked at it in a curious way-
I found three bold labels embossed on its bay.
'God inside' is the first one embossed on the forehead,
Without God's soul, the body would be there but dead.
What gives the body life, vivacity and current is the soul,
You are a living, intelligent, divine being because of the soul.
'Heart inside' is embossed on the mid-chest,
Take tender loving care or it might get upset.
Human beings must be dealt with lovingly and tenderly,
Or else the emotions inside may get hurt suddenly.
'Animal inside' is the third label on the mid-abdomen,
Beware! May be dangerous! Take care or face problems.
The animal within can cross the limits of cruelty,

For self preservation and territory it may abandon all charity.
This strange mixture, thus is what is man;
Divinity, beauty and ugliness you may see all in one man!
Knowing thus we handle ourselves and others with care,
So that we may not bring anyone to despair!
The animal within each, must each one of us subdue,
The divine being within may then shine through!
If we can curb selfishness and full of love live for others,
The best of human beings is then born within us ***Brother!***

-

THE INVULNERABLE SPIRIT OF MAN

-

Man as we have seen is very vulnerable to the whims of Mother
Nature. But he is also possessed with an indomitable, invulnerable
spirit. That inner strength in the midst of peril is what makes man
a man. This inner power makes him smile and laugh over severe
predicaments that he is often faced with and many a times
overcomes them, be it diseases like cancer or social ailments like
poverty and deprivation. Man is very adjusting, accommodating
creature and has learned to laugh in the midst of trouble.

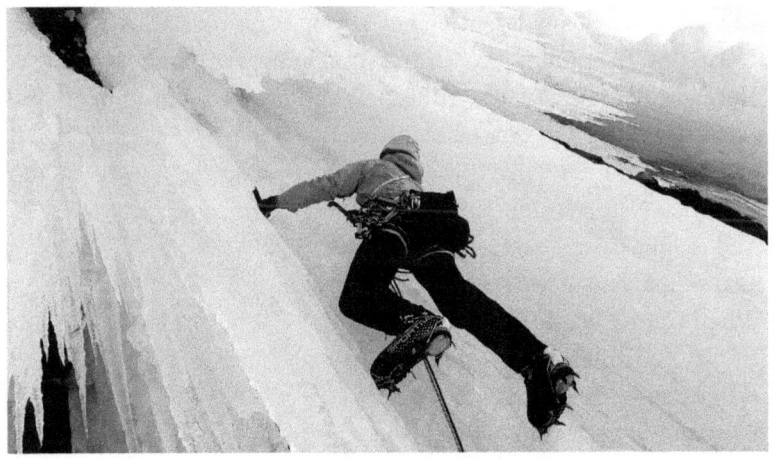

Bravo! That is 'The Spirit!'

<u>That's the Spirit!</u>
Life will sometimes knock you tight,
Lob you left, center and to the right.
Flatten you; smother you in the fight,
You'll be beaten and roughed up in daylight.
Aptly called, "the University of Hard Knocks,"
Life'll make your boat severely tilt and rock.
Life will play these games with you O dear,
It'll chide you, mock you and lay you bare.
Will you cry, be afraid, depressed or withdrawn?
Curse life with your every breath and yawn?
Or will you be able to keep your calm and cool,
Know life's purpose in using knocks as a tool.
Have you prepared yourself for some knocks?
Gathered enough mental strength in your stock--
Thoughts of strength, vigour and invincibility of Spirit.
Of courage and belief in ultimate victory of your grit.
Knocks are a way of teaching us lessons,
To make us strong so our weaknesses lessen.
Let's take the due knocks with a mental poise,
Smile at the naughty, often belligerent ways of life!
P.S. At this point the author remembers a poem by Angela
Morgan (1875-1957). It is called, 'When nature wants a man'. It is
written in 1918, the year of Spanish Flu pandemic. It is a long poem.
Its first few lines go like this:
When Nature wants to drill a man
And thrill a man,
And skill a man,
When Nature wants to mould a man
To play the noblest part;
When she yearns with all her heart
To create so great and bold a man
That all the world shall praise-

Watch her method, watch her ways!
How she ruthlessly perfects
Whom she royally elects;
How she hammers him and hurts him
And with mighty blows converts him
Into trial shapes of clay which only Nature understands-
The full poem can be read at: https://www.poemhunter.com/poem/when-nature-wants-a-man/comments/

-

A DOCTOR IS FOR THE WHOLE WORLD

-

A doctor while growing in physical age grows also in experience, maturity and understanding. He starts to find unity in the midst of all the visible diversity. He comes to recognize that differences are all superficial; deep down there is Unity of Man. Men may believe deeply in their differences but the doctor cannot reasonably hold on to the differences between people, differences of all types that he is bombarded with. All differences get flattened out when they see a doctor or when a doctor sees them.

-

Beyond this and that......
Being a doctor, all my life I traveled far and wide,
I practiced my art in several nations globe-wide.
I treated patients everywhere; no one asked my creed,
I treated them same way, beyond color, religion or creed.
I lived in a locality and we had all kinds of neighbors,
We helped each other in need and lived like brothers.
I didn't know my neighbors' religion, nor they my creed,
We lived beyond all these, we lived through our deeds.
When I was a student, our class was international and huge,
We made friends with everyone, there was such a deluge.
With friends, who bothers religion and who bothers creed?
Friendship is heart to heart, beyond religion as well as creed.
When you see a thing of art, it is beyond this or that,
When science progresses, it benefits all beyond this or that.

Floods, earthquakes, tsunamis don't care for your this or that,
The great equalizer in the end comes to all beyond this or that.
Happiness and sadness have no religion or creed,
They affect all, across borders of cast and creed.
In fact there is nothing that divides us, do pay heed,
Humans can't be divided through color, religion or creed.
Take example of nations, each depends on every other,
Nations are bound by inter-dependence like unknowing brothers.
Humans are a family that can't be divided by this or that,
Divisions and differences are superficial, unity is deeper than all that!

-

UNITY OF MANKIND

-

No one knows it better than a doctor. A doctor has observed the unity of mankind at close quarters, day in and day out. He can't be fooled. Leave everything apart, we breathe the same air, all of us and all of us can't survive without it for 2,3 or say four minutes. As if that was not enough for unification, we are born and die the same way despite our adopted, ingrained and hardened differences that we believed and are stuck with. We all come from The Great Unknown and go back to the same Great Unknown-all of us without exception. We must assert the unity of mankind and refuse to hold on to all differences which in the last analysis are superficial and inconsequential.

-

A & E

In the hospital I worked there was a department called A&E,
Accident and emergency department was known as A&E.
Today what I talk of is a different universal kind of A&E,
Wherever your eyes go you will find these two, the A&E.
Whatever you see has two components called A and E,
A stands for Appearance and E for Essence in our A&E!
Take anything whatever, it has both A and E,

There is an appearance and there is the essence; all is A&E.

Go to Gold market, you see bangles, necklaces, rings and crowns,

These are all appearances; essence is gold if you break them down.

You go to the beach and see waves big and small, slow and fast,

The waves of the ocean are appearances; water is the essence in fact.

Soft snow, liquid water, solid ice or steam; water is their essence in all they seem,

Bubbles of different sizes and colors; air is the essence, bubbles give it a gleam.

Human bodies of different colors, shapes and sizes what is their essence?

Its food, water, air, space, mind, energy and the spirit; that's the common essence!

Whatever and wherever you see, see appearance and see the essence,

Often we so get lost in appearance, we forget to see the essence.

You won't get lost in the jungle of appearances if you never missed the essence,

Appearances are diverse and confusing, what unites us all is the essence.

Why we get lost is because often the essence is hidden and appearance is upfront,

We have to remove the curtain of appearances to see the essence bare and upfront.

It is essential to see the essence and see the unity behind the diverse creation,

Knowing Unity gives peace; diversity is confounding & deceptive, fools us in this creation!

-

Diversity is from Unity

Diversity is so glamorous its pull so great and real,

Variety is so charming; as we follow it, it seems so real.

Like on a sunny day water on the road ahead seems real,

Come close, there is no water only the road is real.
Our outgoing senses are attracted to the charming unreal,
The beauty that pulls you, mind you, is only superficial.
True beauty lies deeper; it created the glam superficial,
See the one behind all; diversity disappears; unity becomes real.
If you keep looking out, variety is great, you'll get lost,
Seek and find unity behind diversity, you'll be saved even if lost.
Turbulence, restlessness, exhaustion come if you follow diversity,
Rest and peace, calm and quiet remain if you can perceive unity.
After every sensory exposure that made diversity look real,
Come home and look deep till you find the basic unity real.
Each day expel diversity and bring unity to the fore,
Or else you're doomed; lost on the surface, far from the core.
In core it's all one, essence of all is one; cause of diversity is one,
One life enlivens all; without life there's nobody, no one.
Keep your eyes on that one; you won't get lost in the bewitching world,
Peace and Joy will be yours; you won't look for them in the outside world.

-

UNITY IS PRIMARY, DIFFERENCES ARE SECONDARY

-

The unity of mankind is beyond doubt, for a doctor. He only wonders at the process of indoctrination which causes the child in everyone to lose his or her innocence which also sees only unity. We breathe the same air, live in the same one space, eat food and drink water from earth, so one. We suffer from same diseases and then one day die. So, one. Why squabble? For beliefs? For concepts? For notions? All acquired through drilling and repetition, not original. Original is innocence, naturalness, human-ness. Just being human!

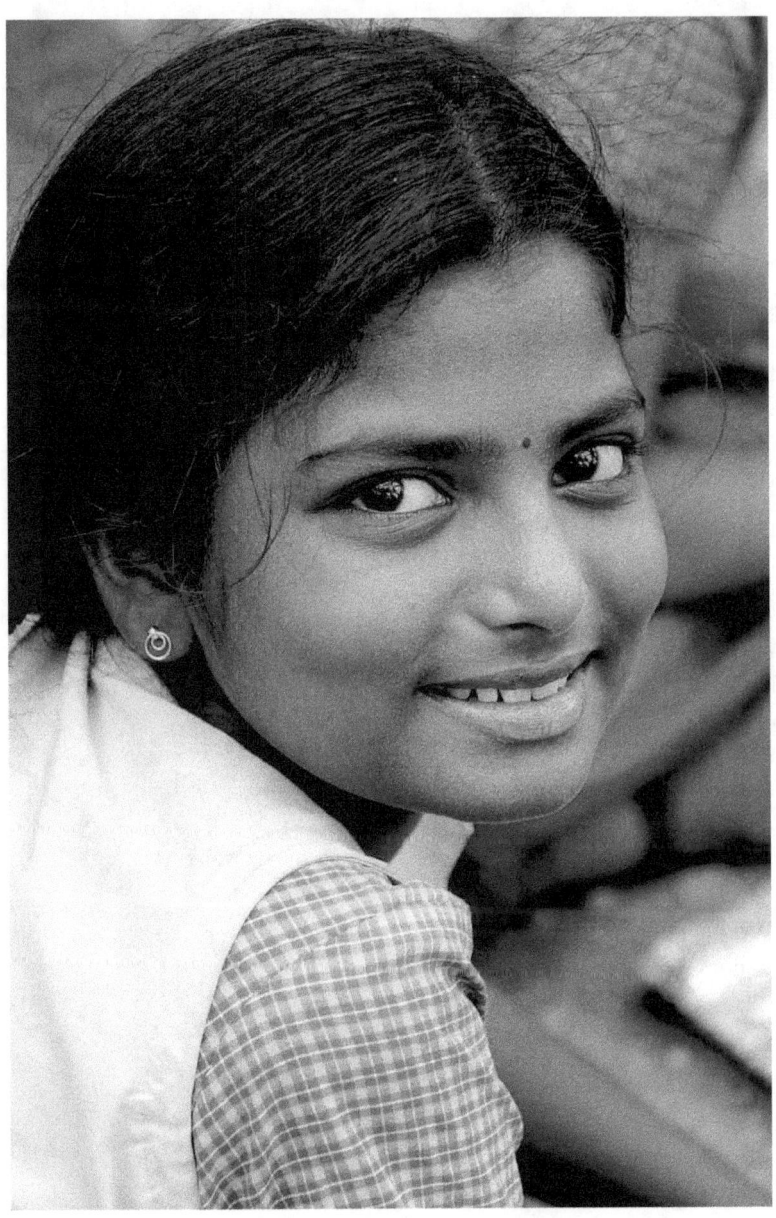

Innocence is intact in a child!

-

Innocence Lost!
When a child comes out of a mother's womb,
And lustily cries,
Can you tell when you hear the cry-
If the baby is black or white,
Muslim, a Jew or a follower of Christ?
You only say,
"Wow! A baby is born!"
When you hear a child's gusty laughter,
In the distance,
A smile or a guffaw enlivens your face,
That contagious laughter touches your soul,
But you can't tell the child's faith,
If he is a Christian or a follower of Islam.
For we are only human when we are born!
Alas! That's when our similarity ends.
Then begins the baptizing and indoctrination,
Differentiation and regimentation!
We create permanent differences in the child's mind,
Through fear, hatred, half-truths, lies and their kind!
A biased and a closed mind is born,
This one looks at the world with particular glasses on!

Very soon the child's innocence is lost,
Oneness disappears; distrust is his lot.
From now it is his belief better than the other,
And then it is one against another.
Humanity cries, humanity suffers!
Good Lord in heavens duly wonders,
I wish they knew 'Me' as well as they thunder."
-

-

-

CHILDREN ARE ANGELS

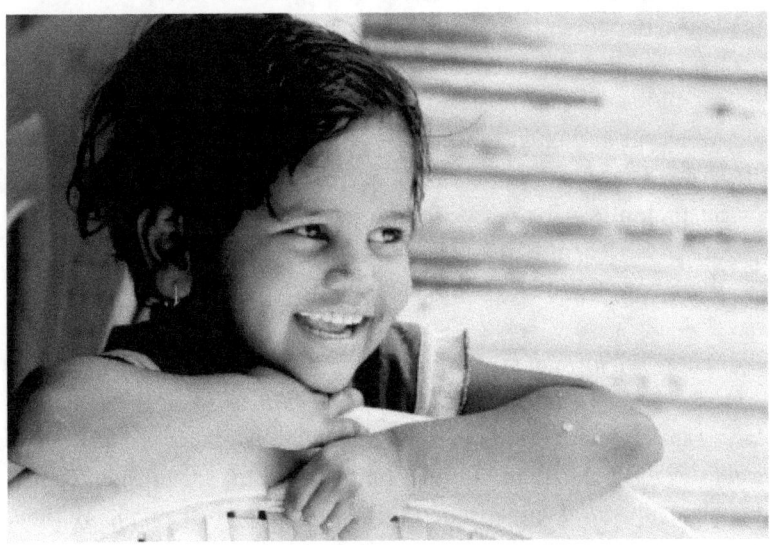

An Angel!

<u>Wish to be a child again!</u>
I sat beside a three year old in a plane,
This Italian child played with his car and a train.
He rolled his car on my sleeve at first,
He thus broke the ice and showed his trust.
I took the lead and became his playmate,
Within minutes we were pals without a debate.
I uttered no words and nor did he,
We had fun and laughter in utter glee.
For the full seven and a half hours of the flight,
From NY to Milan we were friends in delight.
While leaving he smiled and waved a goodbye,
And left an imprint of love on my mind's eye.
We had religious, cultural, language and racial barriers,

The child was pure, unsullied by these unity demolishers.
Simple human to human relations a child knows,
And that's all that we should all be required to know.
These barriers maintain divisions in our one race,
Isn't it abhorring and a disgrace?
A child is the true representative of human race,
All learnt and taught differences are a lot of waste.
How I wish I would be a child again!
Suspicion-less, hate-less, free mind will be mine gain.
But these learnt barriers hang heavy around our necks,
We labor all life like bullocks with this yoke on our necks.

-

"There is a form of laughter that springs from the heart, heard every day in the merry voice of childhood, the expression of a laughter — loving spirit that defies analysis by the philosopher, which has nothing rigid or mechanical in it, and totally without social significance. Bubbling spontaneously from the heart of child or man. Without egotism and full of feeling, laughter is the music of life."

William Osler. Two Frenchmen on Laughter. Men and Books. CMAJ 1912;(II):152

-

LAST WORD

We have come a full circle! Man always comes a full circle! His journey begins as a child and ends up like a child, as they say an old man becomes like a child. William Shakespeare when he said, 'Child is the father of man', he probably meant that a child can teach man a lot. Men have a lot to learn from a child. His or her simplicity, honesty, straight forwardness, innocence, non duplicity, spontaneous and this moment living, now crying and soon smiling and laughing are all qualities of a child that we love to emulate. An adult had all this but loses it all in his journey of growing up through struggles of comparison, competition and criticisms. Every adult wants to regain the paradise of childhood lost along the way. When his wisdom matures and he has accumulated enough experiences of life, he is often able to come back to the original child that he so strongly yearns to be. Simplicity and simple living are peace and joy givers. No one can miss or forego them. That is the culmination of wisdom itself, of the journey of life itself. May everyone reach the joy and bliss of life!

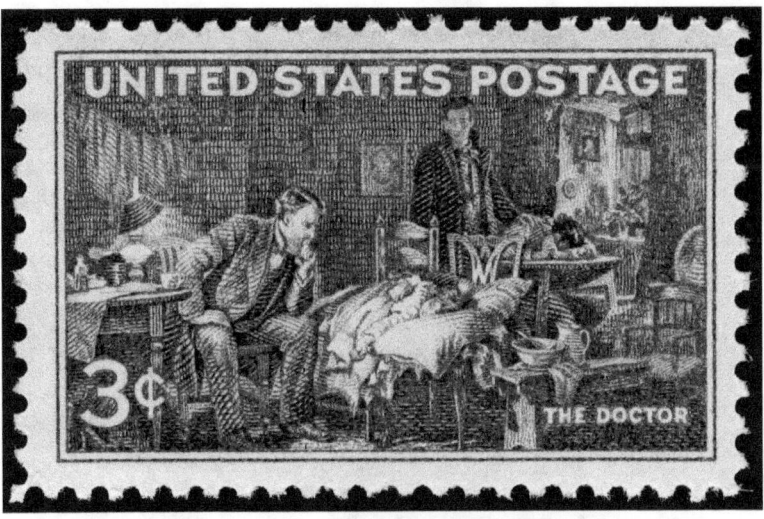

On The American Medical Association Centennial in 1947, US issued a 3 cent stamp depicting 'The Doctor' honoring The Doctors!

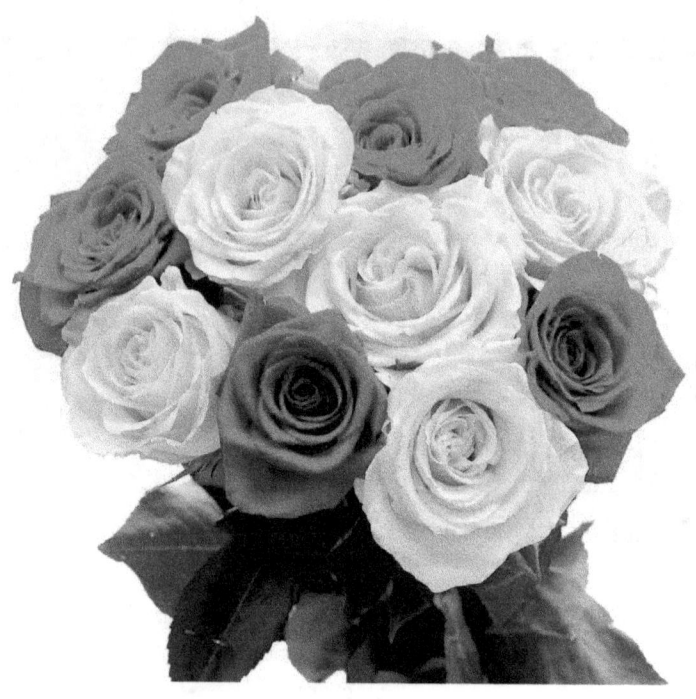

Here is a bouquet of Lovely Roses for Doctors! Thank You!

Author Information

Dr Anil Kumar Chawla did his M.B.B.S from Government Medical College, Rohtak, Haryana, India and was adjudged the best graduate of the class and is a happy member of the ROHMEDICOS 68 fraternity. Following this he did his M.D. in Medicine from the prestigious Post Graduate Institute of Medical Education and Research, Chandigarh, India. He progressed through the stages of Senior Residency in Medicine at the All India Institute of Medical Sciences, New Delhi and Lecturer in Medicine at The A.I.I.M.S New Delhi and Maulana Azad Medical College, New Delhi. He later worked in Oman and Bahrain in various capacities and peaked as Associate Professor of Medicine, Oman Medical College, Sohar, Oman.

He qualified as a Member of the Royal College of Physicians of the United Kingdom and was later elected as a Fellow of the Royal College of Physicians and Surgeons of Glasgow.

During his professional journey he got the opportunity to treat patients of multiple nationalities, teach medicine to students in India and Arab countries and interact with physicians and doctors from India, Arab countries, United Kingdom and United States of America.

He has published scientific papers in national and international journals.

Reading and writing of poetry, art and literature have been his hobbies since high school days. Hindi, English, Urdu, Punjabi are the languages he often delves in to and can read and speak Arabic too!

This work is a dedication to the doctors who are serving humanity in this critical period of COVID 19 pandemic devastating the patients as well as their doctors worldwide.

Salutations to all those selfless serving doctors who are putting their lives on the line to save humanity from this deadly and dreaded virus!

References And Image Credits

References for the Preface:

1. Amanda Howe, Peter Campion, Searle, Helen. New perspectives—approaches to medical education at four new UK medical schools. BMJ 5 August 2004,329: 327, 7461,

   2) Medical Schools Council. Guiding principles for the admission of medical students—revised. 2006. www.medschools.ac.uk/Publications/Pages/Guiding-Principles-Medical-Students.aspx

3. Coulehan Jack, Clary Patrick. Healing the healer: Poetry in palliative care. Journal of Palliative Medicine. Volume 8, No.2, 2005.
4. Williams WC: Asphodel, that greeny flower. In: Selected Poems, New York: New Directions, 1985, p 302
5. McManus IC. Humanity and the medical humanities. Lancet 1995; 346: 1143-45.
6. Barnard D. Making a place for the humanities in residency education. Acad Med 1994; 69: 628-30.
7. American Board of Internal Medicine. Evaluation of humanistic qualities in the internist. Ann Intern Med 1983; 99: 720-24.
8. Association of American Medical Colleges. Report of the working group on personal qualities, values, and attitudes: physicians in the twenty-first century. J Med Educ 1984; 59 (suppl): 177-89.
9. Charon R, Trautmann Banks J, Connelly JE, et al. Literature and medicine: contributions to clinical practice. Ann Intern Med 1995; 122: 599-606.
10. Arnold RM, Povar GJ, Howell JD. The humanities, humanistic behavior, and the humane physician; a cautionary note. Ann Intern Med 1987; 106: 313-18.

11. Povar GJ, Keith KJ. The teaching of liberal arts in internal medicine residency training. J Med Educ 1984; 59: 714-21.

12. Stony Brook University

13. Horowitz, Harold W., Poetry on rounds: A model for the integration of humanities into residency training. Lancet, 2/17/96, Vol. 347, Issue 8999

14. William Foster, Elaine Freeman. Poetry in general practice education: perception of learners. Family Practice(2008) 25 (4): 294-303

15. Green JP. Physicians practicing other occupations especially literature. Mt Sinai J Medicine; 1983 Mar; 60 (2): 132-55

16. Jones, Anne Hudson. Literature and Medicine: Physician poets. Lancet 1997; 349: 275-78

17. Bryant DC. A roster of twentieth-century physicians writing in English. Lit Med 1994; 13: 284-305.

IMAGE CREDITS

All pictures are taken from Google images; most through advanced search for Copyright free, 'free for reuse even commercially' images. Some of these images are from Wikimedia Commons and free to use and are mentioned to be in Public Domain for reasons given. Some of them are from other free image sites like Pixabay, pxfuel etc free images source and some have the Creative Commons license which allows free use of images with attribution.

The individual credits are given below with profuse thanks from the author.

DEDICATION

1. The Doctor : By Joseph Tomanek, reproduction of original painting by Luke Fildes - http://resource.nlm.nih.gov/101394138, Public Domain, https://commons.wikimedia.org/wiki/File: The _Doctor_Joseph_Tomanek_after_Luke_Fildes.jpg https://commons.wikimedia.org/w/index.php?curid=422613

FOREWORD: CONSECRATION

2. Sir William Osler on ward rounds at John Hopkins, Baltimore. Credit: Wellcome Library, London. Wellcome Images. images@wellcome.ac.uk http://wellcomeimages.orgSir William Osler on ward round at Johns Hopkins Hospital in Baltimore, USA. Copyrighted work available under Creative Commons Attribution only license CC BY 4.0 https://creativecommons.org/licenses/by/4.0/

Ref. PP/WRO. The slide illustrates a lecture given by Oliver Wrong ('Osler and My Father') which was based on his article of the same name in the Journal of the Royal Society Medicine 2003 September; 96(9): 462-464. Photograph c. 1889-1905 PP/WRO Professor

Sir William Osler quotes: https://litfl.com/eponymictionary/oslerisms/

CHAPTER 1

1. Student studying, head behind books : https://www.pikist.com/free-photo-soufa
2. Science: The Alchemist. Painting by David Teniers the younger, between 1640 and 1650.

This is a faithful photographic reproduction of a two-dimensional, public domainwork of art. The work of art itself is in the public domain for the following reason:

This work is in the **public domain**in its country of origin and other countries and areas where the copyright termis the author's **life plus 100 years or fewer.** This file has been identified as being free of known restrictions under copyright law, including all related and neighboring rights.The official position taken by the Wikimedia Foundation is that *"faithful reproductions of two-dimensional public domain works of art are public domain"*.

3. **File: Flying Seagull (2704154711).jpg** https://commons.wikimedia.org/wiki/

File:Flying_Seagull_(2704154711).jpg

From Wikimedia Commons, the free media repository.
Western Gull Larus occidentalis, San Diego, California. 22 July 2008, Flying Seagull. Author: Rennett Stowe from USA
This file is licensed under the Creative CommonsAttribution 2.0 Genericlicense.
You are free to share and to remix with attribution and link to the license and say that no changes are made.
4. Close up of seagull
https://www.goodfreephotos.com/animals/birds/close-up-seagull-in-flight-full-wingspan.jpg.php
Free photo of Close-up seagull in flight full wingspan.

All free photos on this site are public domain. Please consider giving a credit hyperlink to https://www.goodfreephotos.com if you use the photos on this site using the attribution code in the below box. It is not required but it'd be much appreciated.
Photo via (https://www.goodfreephotos.com/) Good Free Photos
5. The threshold; Women's high jump at the Triton invitational 2011 at University of California, San Diego. 23 April 2011. Flickr: High Jump Triton Invitational 2011. SD Dirk
This image, which was originally posted to Flickr, was uploaded to Commons using Flickr upload boton 16 August 2012 by Badseed. On that date, it was confirmed to be licensed under the terms of the license indicated. This file is licensed under the Creative CommonsAttribution 2.0 Genericlicense. You are free to share and to remix with attribution and link to the license and say that no changes are made.
6. Tools: Library scene: https://www.pxfuel.com/en/free-photo-jsozx/Free for commercial use.
7. The Anatomy hall: https://commons.wikimedia.org/wiki/File:Iraq._(Mesopotamia).
_Royal_College_of_Medicine_of_Iraq._Baghdad._Medical

College.

The_dissecting_room_LOC_matpc.16043.jpg

From Wikimedia Commons, the free media repository.

Title: Iraq. (Mesopotamia). Royal College of Medicine of Iraq. Baghdad. Medical College. The dissecting room

Abstract/medium: G. Eric and Edith Matson Photograph Collection

Physical description: 1 negative : 1932. Library of Congress.

Catalog: https://www.loc.gov/pictures/collection/matpc/item/mpc2010001540/PP

Original URL: https://hdl.loc.gov/loc.pnp/matpc.16043

No known restrictions on publication.

8. The Robot: https://commons.wikimedia.org/wiki/File:Nao_Robot_(Robocup_2016).jpg

Nao Robot (Robocup2016), 5 July 2016, Own work of Author: ubahnverleih

This file is made available under the Creative CommonsCC0 1.0 Universal Public Domain Dedication

9. Laughing Buddha from Pxfuel; free for commercial use. https://www.pxfuel.com/en/free-photo-qdvti

10. A Young male doctor cartoon

https://pixabay.com/vectors/boy-cartoon-checkup-clinic-comic-2027768/

CHAPTER 2

1. Doctor in the clinic with patient and mother: https://www.pinterest.co.uk/pin/337910778274491107/

2. Sleepy doctor: http://fnews47.blogspot.com/2011/05/dangers-of-lack-of-sleep-in-doctors.html. Posted by Mohammad Nur. Forty Seventh News Monday, 30 May, 2011. Dangers of lack of sleep in doctors.

3. Sherlock Holmes and Dr Watson. https://commons.wikimedia.org/w/index.php?curid=3081229

Watson reading bad news to Holmes in "The Five Orange Pips". One of Sidney Paget's iconic illustrations from *The Strand*magazine. Sydney Paget (1860-1908)- Strand Magazine, appeared in November 1891. Permission details: Public domain: Public Domain

CHAPTER 3

1. Medical insignia: http://clipart-library.com/clipart/gieode5BT.htm
2. The Doctor examining a patient

Dr. Peter Pinto with the Urologic Oncology Branch at the National Cancer Institute (NCI) examines an African-American adult male patient, while an attending physician (male Asian) observes. National Cancer Institute. 3 August 2005.

This image was released by the National Cancer Institute, an agency part of the National Institutes of Health, with the ID 4555(image) (next). See Commons: Licensing.

3. Busy Doctor: from an article: 3 tips to boost your productivity without busting your work-life balance

Jonathan Ford Hughes,*for MDLinx*|November 21, 2018. https://www.mdlinx.com/article/3-tips-to-boost-your-productivity-without-busting-your-work-life-balance/lfc-3010

4. Doctor advising a patient - https://media.gettyimages.com/photos/doctor-explaining-prescription-to-senior-patient-picture-id529114228?b=1&k=6&m=529114228&s=612x612&w=0&h=fd2ukZRD8-5zDIJ2yqMPrDAxSy_yQR462HCc63uXpyY=

5. Doctor with young patient and balloon: "02710009"by IAEA Image bankis licensed under CC BY-SA 2.0. A doctor on the health team prepares to examine a child in Chernobyl, Ukraine, 1990-91.

6. Doctor smoking: https://commons.wikimedia.org/wiki/File:Doctor,_cigarette,_smoking,_stove,_map,_papers_Fortepan_4628.jpg

From Wikimedia Commons, the free media repository

http://www.fortepan.hu/_photo/download/ fortepan_9386.jpgarchive copy

FOTO:Fortepan — ID 4628: Adományozó/Donor: Unknown.Archive copy

The release at fortepan.hu is CC-BY-SA-3.0. As the photographer is unknown or pseudonymous, and the photograph is 85 years old, it is considered public domain both in the country of publication, Hungary, and the USA where Wikimedia Commons is hosted. See Fortepan.HUfor more information on related uploads.

7. Patients waiting in doctor's office: https://commons.wikimedia.org/wiki/File:CCBRT_Disability _Hospital_waiting_room_1_(10679012155).jpg

This file is licensed under the Creative CommonsAttribution 2.0 Genericlicense.

You are free to use, to remix with attribution to the link.

8. The Hospital Bed: https://www.flickr.com/photos/ breadfortheworld/22318750301is licensed under CC BY-ND 2.0Copy. A young patient has his vital signs checked at the San Juan de Dios Hospital, Guatemala. Maria Fleischman/World Bank

9. Christ Among The Doctors: A painting by Jusepe de Ribera(1591-1652)

https://en.wikipedia.org/wiki/ Christ_among_the_Doctors_(D%C3%BCrer)

This is a faithful photographic reproduction of a two-dimensional, public domainwork of art. The work of art itself is in the public domain for the following reason:

The author died in 1652, so this work is in the **public domain**in its country of origin and other countries and areas where the copyright termis the author's **life plus 100 years or fewer**.

This file has been identified as being free of known restrictions under copyright law, including all related and neighboring rights.

10. The Four Doctors of the Western Church https://commons.wikimedia.org/wiki/ File:Gerard_Seghers_(attr)_- _The_Four_Doctors_of_the_Western_Church,_Saint_Jerome.jpg

CHAPTER 4

1. Poor homeless man.

2. Sad Old man. https://pxhere.com/en/photo/924660

3. Taking care of the elderly:

Woman's Mission, Comfort of Old Age, a painting by George
Elgar Hicks.(1824-1914). Tate Britain, London.

under copyright law, including all related and neighboring rights.

The official position taken by the Wikimedia Foundation is that *"faithful reproductions of two-dimensional public domain works of art are public domain"*.

4. Boy and girl smiling: Children's rights. https://www.pikist.com/free-photo-siolu

5. Baby for immunization: Album: Medical Science. Usage: Public domain(CC0), Author: James Gathany, Judy Schmidt, USCDCP/ https://pixnio.com/science/medical-science/immunization-of-children-in-doctors-office

6. Obesity https://www.eatingdisorderhope.com/blog/obesity-binge-eating-disorder-statistics--- CC0 Public Domain. Free for personal and commercial use. No attribution required.

7. Food pyramid: https://www.freepik.com/free-vector/food-pyramid-template-concept_7656741.htm

   Attribution: (https://www.freepik.com/vectors/food) Food vector created by freepik - www.freepik.com

8. Man jogging on the beach https://www.pikist.com/free-photo-vwlsz

9. Waist: Waist/fitness/sport. CC0 Public Domain. Free for personal and commercial use. No attribution required

10. Alopecia areata: Own work by Thirunavukkarasye-Raveendran. 14 July 2017

    https://commons.wikimedia.org/wiki/File:Alopecia_areata_2.jpg
    This file is licensed under the
    Creative CommonsAttribution 4.0International license.
    You are free to share and to remix with attribution and link to the license
    and say that no changes are made.

11. Gas factory: https://www.pxfuel.com/en/free-photo-qbndn/Free for commercial use

12. Angina:

An illustration of a man feeling tightness or pain in the chest - a symptom of angina or of a heart attack. 16 August 2019. https://www.myupchar.com/en/disease/angina

This work is freeand may be used by anyone for any purpose. If you wish to use this content,you do not need to request permission as long as you follow any licensing requirements mentioned on this page.

Wikimedia Foundation has received an e-mail confirming that the copyright holder has approved publication under the terms mentioned on this page.

13. No smoking cartoon: https://pixabay.com/vectors/no-smoking-no-smoking-sign-warning-43907/Pixabay License/Free for commercial use/ No attribution required

14. Pub: https://pixabay.com/photos/pub-bar-drink-london-tap-beer-2243488/

Pixabay License/ Free for commercial use/ No attribution required

15. Drug addiction https://theinscribermag.com/importance-of-primary-care-for-drug-addiction/

Vivek Singh: Vivek is a pro-level blogger with years of experience in writing for multiple industries. He has extensive knowledge in healthcare, business, sports, fashion, and many other popular niches. Vivek has graduated in computer science and has keen interest in traveling. Connect me on Gmail.

16. Road accident: From Wikimedia Commons, the free media repository: https://commons.wikimedia.org/wiki/

17.Road rage: https://commons.wikimedia.org/wiki/File:Road_rage.jpg

-

CHAPTER 5

1. Diogenes- the Greek philosopher: Based on Wikipedia content that has been reviewed, edited and republished, original image by Wikipedia user Singinglemon. Uploaded by Mark Cartwright, published on 02 August 2014 under the following domain: Public Domain. This item is in the public domain and can be used, copied, and modified without any restrictions. https://en.wikipedia.org/wiki/Diogenes

2. Religious symbols: http://www.schoolchalao.com/basic-education/show-results/introduction-of-indian-culture/religions-and-religious-symbols

3. Tsunami Japanese https://www.theatlantic.com/photo/2016/03/5-years-since-the-2011-great-east-japan-earthquake/

473211/a tsunami reaches Miyako City, overtopping seawalls and flooding streets in Iwate Prefecture, Japan, after the magnitude 9.0 earthquake struck the area March 11, 2011. #Mainichi Shimbun / Reuters

4. Three skeletons: Free for commercial use

   https://www.pikrepo.com/fpxya/grayscale-photo-of-human-skull

5. The Fetus :Lunar caustic : Embryo week 9-10 https://www.flickr.com/photos/lunarcaustic/2433149102/in/photostream/

   License: Creative commons--https://creativecommons.org/licenses/by/2.0/

6. The Ice climber.
   https://pixabay.com/photos/ice-climbing-extreme-sports-climb-4000385/Pixabay License. Free for commercial use
   No attribution required
7. Smiling 10 years old girl https://www.pikist.com/free-photo-splol
8. Smiling Innocent child: CC0 Public Domain. Free for personal and commercial use No attribution required. https://pxhere.com/en/photo/596433
9. The Doctor-Stamp by Bureau of Engraving and Printing. - U.S. Postal Service; National Postal Museum: Doctors Issue, Public Domain, https://commons.wikimedia.org/w/index.php?curid=47421039Doctors AMA Centennial 3 cent 1947 issue US stamp, commemorating 100thanniversary of the founding of the American Medical Association. 9 June 1947, US Postal Service, National Postal Museum. Doctors issue, Bureau of Engraving and Printing. Creative commons license.

10. A bunch of red and yellow roses can be had at https://www.cakegift.in/15-red-yellow-roses-bunch